"This book is a gift to all mothers, but more importantly, a gift to all the children of our collective future. A woman's body is the soil in which a new life grows and flourishes. Cleansing, nourishing, supporting, and healing that soil is what Mama Glow *is all about—before, during, and after—so that our next generation of children will be bright, focused, fit, and engaged. If you want to have a baby, or know anyone about to have a baby, this book will save two lives—mother and baby!"*

— **Mark Hyman, M.D.,** author of the #1 *New York Times* bestseller
The Blood Sugar Solution

*"*Mama Glow *reveals the extraordinary power of natural, plant-based living during pregnancy. It is a must-have guide for healthy mothers and their babies."*

— **Neal Barnard, M.D.,** best-selling author of *Food for Life* and
Dr. Neal Barnard's Program for *Reversing Diabetes*

"In Mama Glow, *Latham Thomas delivers an empowering promise of what women would actually like to expect while expecting: a glowing, energetic, and healthy experience that doesn't bring life to a screeching halt. Latham shows us how to feel great and look fantastic, all the while easing our wonky fears about motherhood."*

— **Tara Stiles,** founder of Strala Yoga, best-selling
author of *Yoga Cures* and *Slim Calm Sexy Yoga*

*"*Mama Glow *takes the guesswork out of having a happy pregnancy. It offers a fantastic program for mothers to achieve vitality and ease. I highly recommend it!"*

— **Frank Lipman, M.D.,** founder and director of Eleven Eleven Wellness Center
and author of *Revive: Stop Feeling Spent and Start Living Again*

"I feel blessed to have Latham Thomas on my speed dial. The moment I get pregnant, Latham will be the first call I make. Her holistic approach to pregnancy guides women through the process with joy and confidence. Every woman deserves the miracle of Mama Glow.*"*

— **Gabrielle Bernstein,** author of *May Cause Miracles*

"Latham is an incredible doula. She helped to guide me on the most important journey of my life—welcoming my son into the world. She empowers you so that you are free to focus on welcoming your baby into the world. This book is Latham's gift to women who want to feel that natural glow power."

— **Rebecca Minkoff,** fashion designer

*"*Mama Glow *is the essential handbook for expectant mothers who want to create a peaceful life for themselves and their babies. Latham's passion for helping women become mothers in the most holistic way possible is deeply inspiring."*

— **Joshua Rosenthal,** Founder and Director of the Institute for Integrative Nutrition

"Latham Thomas is convinced that pregnancy is the time for a woman to shine more than ever. In Mama Glow, *she shows every willing mom-to-be how to grow into her most luminous self, before the baby comes and forever after."*

— **Victoria Moran,** author of *Main Street Vegan*

MAMA
GLOW

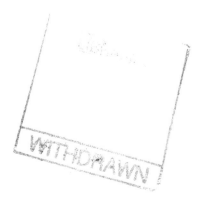

MAMA GLOW

A Hip Lifestyle Guide to Your Fabulous Abundant Pregnancy

LATHAM THOMAS

HAY HOUSE

Australia • Canada • Hong Kong • India
South Africa • United Kingdom • United States

First published and distributed in the United Kingdom by:

Hay House UK Ltd, 292B Kensal Rd, London W10 5BE. Tel.: (44) 20 8962 1230; Fax: (44) 20 8962 1239. www.hayhouse.co.uk

Published and distributed in the United States of America by:

Hay House, Inc., PO Box 5100, Carlsbad, CA 92018-5100. Tel.: (1) 760 431 7695 or (800) 654 5126; Fax: (1) 760 431 6948 or (800) 650 5115. www.hayhouse.com

Published and distributed in Australia by:

Hay House Australia Ltd, 18/36 Ralph St, Alexandria NSW 2015. Tel.: (61) 2 9669 4299; Fax: (61) 2 9669 4144. www.hayhouse.com.au

Published and distributed in the Republic of South Africa by:

Hay House SA (Pty), Ltd, PO Box 990, Witkoppen 2068. Tel./Fax: (27) 11 467 8904. www.hayhouse.co.za

Published and distributed in India by:

Hay House Publishers India, Muskaan Complex, Plot No.3, B-2, Vasant Kunj, New Delhi – 110 070. Tel.: (91) 11 4176 1620; Fax: (91) 11 4176 1630. www.hayhouse.co.in

Distributed in Canada by:

Raincoast, 9050 Shaughnessy St, Vancouver, BC V6P 6E5. Tel.: (1) 604 323 7100; Fax: (1) 604 323 2600

Cover design: Christy Salinas
Interior design: Tricia Breidenthal
Interior photos/illustrations: Micaela Ezra
Indexer: Jay Kreider/Index It Now

A catalogue record for this book is available from the British Library.

ISBN 978-1-84850-923-8

Printted and bound in Great Britain by TJ International Ltd, Padstow, Cornwall

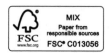

*To my one and only beloved son, Fulano,
who inspires me and keeps me
dialed in to my glow power.*

To my mother and grandmother.

*To you the reader. You have a mandate to glow.
If your eyes have fallen upon these words,
this was meant for you.*

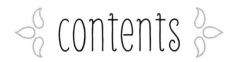

contents

Foreword by Dr. Christiane Northrup　　　　　　　　　　　　　　　　xi
Preface　　　　　　　　　　　　　　　　　　　　　　　　　　　　xiii
Introduction: Your Glow Pilot and How to Navigate This Book　　　　xvii

part I: wellness B.C. (before child)
Chapter 1: The Journey Begins: Ready, Set, GLOW!　　　　　　　　　3
Chapter 2: In the Kitchen: Intro to the Glow Plan　　　　　　　　　15
Chapter 3: On the Mat: Making Clearance　　　　　　　　　　　　37
Chapter 4: In Your Life: Holding the Space　　　　　　　　　　　　45

part II: your abundant pregnancy: first trimester (weeks 1–13)
Chapter 5: The Building Blocks: Baby Steps　　　　　　　　　　　51
Chapter 6: In the Kitchen: Your Prenatal Pantry　　　　　　　　　63
Chapter 7: On the Mat: Prenatal Yoga Principles　　　　　　　　　91
Chapter 8: In Your Life: Sacred Anatomy　　　　　　　　　　　　103

part III: get your glow on!: second trimester (weeks 14–28)
Chapter 9: A Bun in the Oven: Now You're Cookin'　　　　　　　　109
Chapter 10: In the Kitchen: Conscious Cooking and Eating for the Glow　123
Chapter 11: On the Mat: Glowing with the Flow!　　　　　　　　　135
Chapter 12: In Your Life: Glow Potion Beauty Essentials　　　　　　145

part IV: it's glow time!: third trimester (weeks 29–40)
Chapter 13: The Home Stretch: Glow Zone　　　　　　　　　　　157
Chapter 14: In the Kitchen: Comfort Foods　　　　　　　　　　　171
Chapter 15: On the Mat: Tune Out to Tune In　　　　　　　　　　177
Chapter 16: In Your Life: Your Blissful Birth　　　　　　　　　　185

part V: wellness A.D. (after delivery)
Chapter 17: Postpartum and Mama-Glow Mojo: Groovin' Your New Abundant Life　213
Chapter 18: In the Kitchen: Boob Foods　　　　　　　　　　　　231
Chapter 19: On the Mat: Claiming Your New Body　　　　　　　　243
Chapter 20: In Your Life: You *Glow* Girl!　　　　　　　　　　　247

Conclusion　　　　　　　　　　　　　　　　　　　　　　　　　251
Appendix A: Quick Reference Chart of Glow Foods and Super Glow Foods　253
Appendix B: Mama Glow Recipes　　　　　　　　　　　　　　　255
Appendix C: Mama Glow Resources　　　　　　　　　　　　　　305
Appendix D: Blissful Birth Plan　　　　　　　　　　　　　　　313
Conversion Tables　　　　　　　　　　　　　　　　　　　　　318
Index　　　　　　　　　　　　　　　　　　　　　　　　　　　321
Acknowledgments　　　　　　　　　　　　　　　　　　　　　331
About the Author　　　　　　　　　　　　　　　　　　　　　333

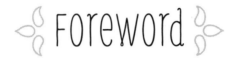

Foreword

Christiane Northrup, MD
author of *Women's Bodies, Women's Wisdom*

Yesterday I was at the hairdressers', when one of the stylists showed me a video of her toddler "playing" at coloring her mama's hair. What was so striking about the video was that this tiny girl knew exactly how to handle her mother's hair—picking up sections in precisely the way all competent stylists do. Then she went into the kitchen and came back with a bowl—the same kind of bowl that her mother used to hold the color she would put on a client's hair. As it turns out, in the last month of her pregnancy, the stylist had worked long hours trying to get all her clients in before she went into labor. And this left an indelible—and adorable—imprint on the daughter in her womb.

I spent many years assisting women in their pregnancies and births, all the while acutely aware of how sacred, precious, and important the events surrounding pregnancy and birth really are. Starting from the very moment you decide to prepare your body for pregnancy, to the moment your baby comes into the world, you are setting the stage for the most intimate relationship of your life: the one between you and your child. And you are also creating the foundation of your baby's health for the rest of his or her life, because the prenatal environment has the power to turn genes—and disease potential down the road—on or off. For example, an undernourished mother will turn on the hunger genes of her child—and those so-called thrifty genes will, in turn, be passed down to that child's children, and even his or her grandchildren! Just like the toddler who emerged from the womb knowing how to color hair, all babies are left with a similar blueprint for their own potential that is largely determined by a mother's diet, thoughts, environment, relationships, fears, hopes, and dreams.

And that is why I am so thrilled with Latham Thomas and her Mama Glow approach to pregnancy and birth. For starters, she begins with her own uplifting and inspiring birth story, which stands in such sharp and lovely contrast to the usual war stories that pregnant women hear every day: how awful labor is, why drugs are necessary, and how much easier it'd be to have a C-section. Our collective emergency mind-set around birth has led to an astounding and dangerous C-section rate of 30 to 50 percent in most major hospitals, despite the fact that a C-section results in four times the maternal death rate of a vaginal birth. Further, the rate of prematurity from inductions done between 37 and 38 weeks has resulted in an estimated $1 billion of additional costs to the health-care system from increased morbidity to mother and baby, intensive-care admissions, and neonatal deaths. If all of this medical intervention actually improved the health of mothers and babies, that would be one thing. But the U.S. spends more money on health care per capita than any nation on earth, and it ranks number 41 in infant mortality worldwide—behind Cuba, Estonia, and Poland! And this ranking has fallen significantly in the last 20 years—closely paralleling the unprecedented rise in birth interventions. But there's more to it than the medical system—just the obesity epidemic alone has also resulted in many more pregnancy complications than in years past. And there's also the fact that 50 percent of pregnancies in the U.S. are still unplanned. Given that infant and maternal mortality are tried and true measures of the health of a nation, it's clear that something needs to change! Fortunately, that change is right in your hands.

There's a light at the end of this grim obstetrical tunnel—a *glow*, actually. And that *glow* is Latham Thomas—and her conscious, uplifting, and hip approach to natural pregnancy and birth. She is part of a generation of young mamas who are bringing sexy back. Sexy health, sexy body, sexy consciousness. This delightful and pleasurable change in consciousness—as well as a fierce ownership of our own bodies and birth magic—is precisely what it's going to take to turn pregnancy and birth back into the sacred life passages they truly are. And put an end to the unnecessary suffering of millions of mothers and babies who simply didn't know any better. Alice Walker once said, "Nothing is more important than how we are born." I agree wholeheartedly. And that's why *Mama Glow* is one of the most important books that you are ever likely to read. Its wisdom will reverberate in your baby's genes for generations.

❧ preface ❧

Under a fierce full moon, on a steamy summer evening in 2003, I was sitting listening to the gospel cries of Mahalia Jackson in my teensy Chelsea apartment, when my water broke. I realized at that moment—as I gathered up my petite belly, gazing down at my soon-to-be-born bundle—that I was about to finally meet my baby. Elated and overwhelmed, I phoned my mom and other family members, my friends, and my midwife to share the news. But really, all I could think was, *Holy shit! I'm about to give birth in a few hours, and I don't have a single diaper in this house!*

I'm a Bohemian-chic, tree-hugging, shoe-loving, urban, vegan vixen and holistic wellness maven living in New York City. When I became pregnant in 2002, I quickly realized that my pregnancy was nothing like those described in the books I was reading. I didn't experience the laundry list of ailments or the drastic physical changes that professional sources claim are "the norm" during pregnancy. In fact, I was comfortable and active throughout, working until the week my son, Fulano, was born. I gained a mere 14 pounds, which melted off after delivery. I never had a day of morning sickness, or even the slightest bit of swelling in my hands, ankles, or feet. (Thankfully so, because I had recently bought some Italian boots that I wasn't prepared to part with.) Instead, I had an abundant and affirming pregnancy and also experienced an ecstatic natural labor and drug-free birth that lasted just four hours, attended by a fantastic nurse-midwife, two nurse assistants, and one intern.

Reflecting on my pregnancy and birth experience, I attributed the ease and comfort to my healthy diet, lifestyle, and attitude. Sure, genetics play a part, but every birth is different, and so is every person. My diet of organic foods and globally inspired vegan cuisine provided me with the necessary nutrients and energy I needed to sustain a healthy pregnancy while feeling good and looking great. My yoga practice was my saving grace. I learned how to tune in to what was happening in my body and ease my mind through meditation. Yoga also informed my birth ritual from beginning to end. I was able to relax into my breathing techniques at the onset of contractions, and I visualized the baby moving farther down the birth canal (which I think of as "the sacred passageway") during each contraction. I knew that every sensation was taking me closer to bringing the baby into the world.

I credit these lifestyle choices and more with giving me what I now call the "Mama Glow." Mama Glow is an abundant, radiant energy that comes from within. Its characteristics include clear and vibrant skin, shining hair, and sparkling eyes. It's about your initiation, birthing yourself as a powerful woman, as you prepare to give birth to your bundle of joy. Birth *is* our rite of passage, and Mama Glow *is* our birthright—to walk in grace, power, and wisdom; to have understanding, reverence, and trust in our bodies. Having faith in the benevolent universe and being an active participant in the co-creation of your fabulous life. This act of standing in your power ignites a force within that glows from the inside out.

Mama Glow comes from a lifestyle plan that includes food, activity, and intention. It starts with eating a balanced diet of locally grown, organic, seasonal, whole foods—"glow foods," as I like to call them—which include power foods like kale, beets, walnuts, cherries, and quinoa, and raw super-foods such as hemp seeds, maca root, and goji berries. In addition to eating, Mama Glow requires adequate exercise, especially yoga, combined with a fulfilling spiritual practice—including empowering affirmations, meditation, and journaling. But even more important, Mama Glow is an attitude—an approach to life, a sense of contentment that reflects a conscious engagement with your pregnancy. *Mama Glow* presents a comprehensive plan for living in the "glow zone" during your pregnancy and beyond: a new way of eating, thinking, exercising, and being. It's a personal style that reflects confidence, beauty, radiance, and balance.

Mama Glow will help you prepare for pregnancy and birth—in the kitchen, on the yoga mat, and in your life. Promoting a plant-based diet of globally inspired vegan cuisine, the pages that follow are filled with an array of tasty recipes that will make you forget all about pickles and ice cream. Peppered with lots of savvy glow tips, *Mama Glow* will help you develop a balanced lifestyle that will have you feeling and looking your very best for the next nine months—and more.

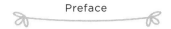

I wrote this book to promote a new type of pregnancy, one that's suited to *you*—the hip, post-*Sex and the City* siren. You're ready to embrace a healthy and holistic lifestyle, what I like to think of as the Soul and the City lifestyle. *Mama Glow* aims to offer you the valuable nutritional, physical, and spiritual guidance you need to get there, regardless of your age or background.

Pregnancy is a perfect time to really get to know yourself—to resolve any personal issues, learn to trust your instincts, learn to trust and love your body, and develop a connection with your unborn baby. It's a time to shine! It's a time to feel beautiful, from the inside out. Put on those swanky sandals and slip into that sultry, form-fitting, spaghetti-strap dress. This is a celebration! You are the center of attention, and your blooming belly gets the spotlight. While your baby grows and expands inside you, you are growing and expanding in consciousness. You are maturing; you're preparing for the biggest trip of your life. You are embodying Mama Glow.

My name is Latham Thomas, and I am the founder of Mama Glow Lifestyle, co-founder of the Mama Glow Film Festival, and the creator of the Mama Glow prenatal lifestyle and yoga technique. I am a certified holistic health coach, green chef, vinyasa yoga instructor, and birth coach. I've worked with hundreds of women in New York City and beyond, helping them prepare for birth and motherhood. I am honored be your "glow pilot" as you journey through this book and your pregnancy—guiding you to incorporate small, everyday changes on your way to a healthier and happier you. My mission is to empower you to take charge of your life by embracing your well-being, developing a healthy relationship with food, and finding spiritual and physical balance in your life, which should be nothing less than absolutely fabulous! So let's fasten our seat belts, put on our aviator shades, and enjoy this wild ride!

Latham Thomas
New York City

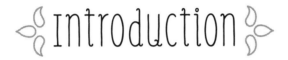

Introduction

Your Glow Pilot and How to Navigate This Book

The total experience of pregnancy involves body, mind, and spirit. This means that our health depends on more than our diet, our genetic makeup, or our environment. That's why this book is chock-full of accessible nutritional information; dietary guidelines; healthy, delicious, globally inspired, plant-based recipes; home remedies; yoga *asanas;* meditations; affirmations; lifestyle tips; anecdotal stories; and an abundance of other resources. If I have my way, by the end of this book, you'll not only feel great but will also have the information you need to take action and harness that beautiful Mama Glow!

My Mama Glow Experience

My journey into motherhood took 290 days—like many first-born babies, my son was a week late. When I became pregnant, I didn't know much about the resources available or the various birthing options. Back then there weren't as many websites and baby blogs churning out helpful information as there are today, and there were only a few organizations helping to navigate birthing options. All I knew was that I was having a baby. I had to get myself together—and fast, honey! And so I did. By the time my son was born, I'd accumulated so much valuable information I not only compiled a book of my own but also began developing courses for expecting mothers and birth educators. Eventually, I founded Tender Shoots Wellness, a boutique lifestyle company for expectant and new moms who want to embrace their pregnancies holistically.

The book you now hold in your hands is an at-home version of the curriculum I offered NYC moms through my Tender Shoots Wellness consulting practice, which is now offered through my company Mama Glow. It contains advice—practical, sensible, ancestral, and in tune with the rhythms of our bodies and those of the little ones growing inside us. It will, I hope, provide you with the tools necessary to make your journey into motherhood as joyful, rich, and fulfilling for you as mine was. Every day, I see this information create tremendous shifts in the women I work with. I see how taking a holistic approach helps them change in their thinking, in their feelings, and in their being—results that, for me, are priceless.

Every mother's experience of birth is unique. Much like the practice of yoga, pregnancy involves a union of mind, body, and spirit. We must align with the source of the divine energy that allows the miracle of life to grow inside us. This energy enables egg and sperm to conjoin and give rise to the complex individual who will be your child. It creates life within you for nine months, and continues past birth in the form of love—the love you feel for your baby, and vice versa. That's some pretty powerful energy, girlfriend!

That's why being pregnant is more than simply bringing another human into the world. It's not a medical condition, and it's more than a simple propagation of the species. It's certainly not a competition—about who can stay the skinniest or look the prettiest, who can do the most Kegel exercises, or who can resist her cravings the longest. It's not about denying things to yourself or setting unrealistic goals. Nor is it about trying to be "the same old you" and do all the things the "old you" did. There is no point in entering into this kind of competition with yourself. There will be no gold medal waiting for you once you deliver the baby! Pregnancy is not about doing it "right"; it's about being open to change, about softening and allowing yourself to surrender to the forces at work within you. A divine energy is cultivating a new life and a new you. Pregnancy therefore presents us with an extraordinary opportunity to become conscious on multiple levels—and brings us to a completely new place within ourselves spiritually.

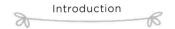

Pregnancy is a transformational event on every level—emotional, physical, and spiritual. We become more flexible in our thinking and in our joints, too. Our senses sharpen, and our tendency to follow gut instinct is more pronounced. We're deeply connected to our changing body and the tiny being sharing space with us. A cocktail of hormones is flooding our bloodstream and preparing us for the main event—the big bang! We may start feeling intensely aware and sensitive to stimuli, and we may feel more grounded physically. Whatever effects we experience, we need an actionable lifestyle plan that helps us stay aligned with the miracle of life happening through us.

How to Navigate This Book

Mama Glow explores a holistic lifestyle approach to pregnancy in the kitchen, on the yoga mat, and in your life. My hope is to support your needs and goals before, during, and after pregnancy—addressing your mind, body, spirit . . . and your inner diva. Yes, I said *diva!* And I mean it in the fiercest sense of the word. A diva is a woman who is claiming her power. A goddess who allows her divine light to shine from within. Throughout the book, I may refer to your inner diva as your goddess guru or simply your glow. It's all the same to me. It means I'm calling on your spirit—the deepest, most intimate part of yourself.

Mama Glow takes you through every stage of pregnancy. We start in Part I, Wellness B.C. (Before Child), where we make clearance for the pregnancy, addressing detox and diet, toxic habits, and incorporating yoga and contemplative practices to get you on track for an awesome pregnancy. Part II focuses on the first trimester, your changing body, common discomforts, stocking your prenatal pantry, Mama Glow yoga principles, and an exploration of sacred anatomy. Part III looks at the second trimester, including finding a health-care provider for your baby, making healthy lifestyle choices that will give your baby the best start, more tasty food and yoga, and some beauty solutions. You'll learn to flow and practice affirmations. We'll also explore sex and birth—two sides of the same coin.

Part IV focuses on the final trimester: preparing for birth, labor coaches, birth plans, yoga postures for comfort, comfort foods, and the anatomy of labor and birth. Part V is the postpartum section. Here I help new moms navigate motherhood—guiding you back to your prebaby body, offering tips for breastfeeding and optimal nutrition, and giving insight on how to step into your new role.

Mama Glow debunks some of the widespread myths and misconceptions around pregnancy. You'll find answers to sensitive questions you may hesitate to

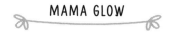
ask a medical professional—for example, *How much weight do I really need to gain? What can I do to keep my digestion regular? After the birth, how do I get back to my prebaby body?* And the all-important question, *What about my sex drive?!* (Vroom, vroom!) You'll find accessible information about yoga and its practical applications for pregnancy, labor, and after birth. *Mama Glow* has the tools necessary for you to enjoy an abundant pregnancy, while giving you information on various support structures every step of the way. You'll learn how to create your "sister circle," a network of women you can count on as you transition into motherhood; you'll discover how to listen to your body and deconstruct your cravings; and you'll find out how to re-integrate your body postpartum. The *Mama Glow* Trimester Checklists will help keep you organized, while a host of helpful practices and techniques will help make the shift to motherhood as comfortable and fulfilling as possible.

Mama Glow also contains tips on how to support your health season by season and how to integrate glow foods into your daily diet. I will introduce you to vegan and raw cuisine, including the philosophy and value of veganism, organics, and sustainable green living. I'll even guide the wannabe mommy through a prepregnancy detox diet plan designed to rid your body of energy-depleting toxins, shed excess weight, gain clarity of focus and peace of mind, and restore your emotional and physical wellness in preparation for pregnancy.

In other words, *Mama Glow* presents a way of eating, thinking, exercising, and *being*. It's about birthing ourselves as mothers—mothering ourselves first—so that we're healthy, willing, and able to give our best to our babies, families, and the world.

In the Kitchen

Our bodies have the remarkable ability to self-heal, ward off illness, and sustain new life. In modern times the efforts that our bodies make to keep us healthy have been undermined by our reliance on denatured and nutrient-depleted foods— what many refer to as SAD, also known as the Standard American Diet. This book shows you how to redress the balance by adding glow foods that stimulate the immune system, balance the hormonal system, and supply the body with the nutrients it needs to promote optimal well-being for you and your baby. These glow foods will be woven throughout the In the Kitchen section of each chapter. Each glow food will be presented with its own nutritional profile, corresponding recipes, and specific ways it can be used to ease common discomforts in particular stages

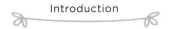

of pregnancy. The recipes are found throughout the book, and there are more recipes for glow meals and meal plans in Appendix B. Think Sweet Lemongrass and Lime Corn. Carrot Cumin Dip. Butternut Squash Apple Soup. Lavender-Ginger Goddess Tonic . . . you get the idea.

Once you understand the simple principles of eating for the glow and start incorporating tasty, health-supportive recipes into your diet, you'll be on your way to increased vitality during pregnancy and beyond. Even better? You'll not only *feel* more energetic—you will notice a difference in the way you *look* as well. (Hey—let's not kid ourselves, it matters!)

On the Mat

Yoga is a wonderful training ground for birth and parenting. It helps cultivate awareness and meditation in daily actions. For this reason, a key component of the Mama Glow prenatal program happens on the yoga mat. But the techniques you will learn in the yoga sections of the book can be applied both on and off the mat. A fruitful Mama Glow yoga practice will foster awareness of the very real connection between mind, body, and spirit. Yoga honors the inner resources and innate wisdom of the body and mind, which is especially important as you prepare for labor and mothering. The dynamic prenatal yoga practice I teach will support your health and well-being throughout pregnancy—as well as prepare you mentally, emotionally, and physically for childbirth.

The Mama Glow yoga technique focuses on affirmations/meditations, *pranayama* (breath work), pregnancy-specific asanas (postures), and alignment that strengthens the body and protects the mobile joints of the expectant mother. This nurturing sequence of postures and exercises requires no previous yoga experience.

Use the Mama Glow principles—Mindfulness, Intention, Flexibility, Tuning Inside, Glow Power, Gratitude, and Opening—which we will visit throughout the book to help guide you in your yoga practice and in your personal life. These principles are an integral part of each On the Mat yoga section and are also worked into the practice exercises in the In Your Life journaling sections at the end of each chapter. Yoga's cultivation of mindfulness and awareness in the moment is the perfect way to begin preparing for this exciting life transformation.

In Your Life

Finding balance in your life requires self-reflection. It means you have to acknowledge your power in creating your circumstances. Only once you are living in full awareness can you facilitate change. The In Your Life sections of *Mama Glow* focus on setting intentions and exploring your challenges, beliefs, goals, and dreams—all the while integrating the Mama Glow principles and engaging in journaling exercises.

During my pregnancy I set an intention to be healthy, stay active until my due date, and have a natural labor. I committed myself to this intention and aligned my actions around fulfilling the agreement I made with myself. Not only did I have a healthy pregnancy, but as I said earlier, I worked until the week I gave birth and had a remarkably swift natural labor.

A big part of my personal time during pregnancy was spent journaling. I used it as a way to record my experiences, and also to track my personal growth. Taking radical responsibility for my life, taking charge of my pregnancy, and mothering myself—in other words, observing the Mama Glow principles—helped me develop confidence, stay present, and operate from a place of joy, gratitude, and abundance. I'm not saying I never had a bad day, and I'm not implying that I'm perfect! What I mean to say is that I internalized my experiences in a totally different way; I was grateful for the challenges and for what those moments could teach me.

The In Your Life sections will ask you to engage in self-inquiry, exploring your own nature and any blocks standing in the way of fulfilling your highest potential. These sections move beyond pregnancy, having to do with your creativity in general. They will help you begin to masterfully co-create the life you want. You'll start to see that life is not happening *to* you, it's happening *through* you. As you physically expand with new life, you are also growing mentally, spiritually, and emotionally. You are preparing for the transformation to motherhood. This is what I want you and all pregnant women to experience: a total embrace of who you are. I hope the In Your Life chapters will help you honor who you are becoming over the course of your journey as both a woman and a mother.

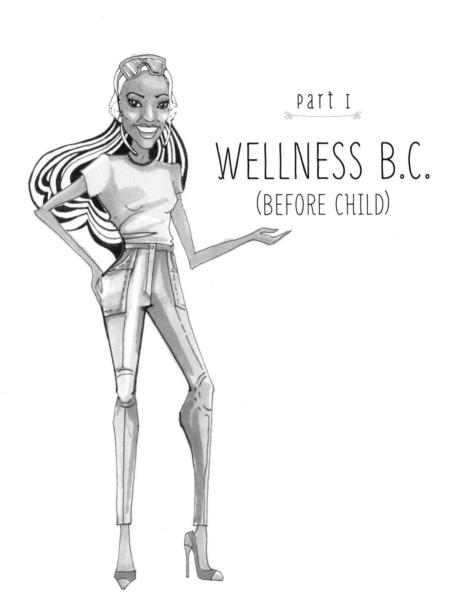

PART I

WELLNESS B.C.
(BEFORE CHILD)

CHAPTER 1

THE JOURNEY BEGINS

Ready, Set, GLOW!

So you want to have a baby? Welcome to a sacred club, my friend. You are embarking on an important mission, and rather than a traditional co-pilot, you are getting me—your personal "glow pilot." I will be your closest confidante throughout your journey, starting here: preparing to get pregnant in the first place.

The goal of this chapter is to get you in a place of physical well-being, spiritual fitness, and emotional balance before you conceive. You will learn to respect your body and how it communicates with you. You will integrate self-care practices on a more regular basis, practices that honor your needs and help grow your glow. It's time to shine, girlfriend!

This chapter is also about putting your life in order and clearing out what no longer belongs—cleaning the slate, so to speak. Why is that important? It's quite simple actually. When you remove what's holding you back in your life (like relationships that no longer work, bad habits like staying up late or excessive drinking or smoking, or too much stress) you create space for your dreams, intentions, and goals—including pregnancy—to come to fruition. We'll do this from the inside out. The first step—and the subject of this chapter—will be a prepregnancy detox. It will enable you to restore your clarity and peace of mind, rid your body of energy-depleting toxins, and shed excess weight. In other words, get ready to take on that fierce Mama Glow I keep talking about. So on your mark, get set, *glow*!

Clearing Out the Clutter

The prepregnancy detox begins where you may least expect: your home. When you have company coming over you don't leave the house a total mess, do you? Ideally you take a little time to tidy up. At the very least, you do a once-over in the bathroom and kitchen. Even better if you do a deep clean—scrub, mop, wax, and sweep.

Your home is not only a reflection of who you are on the outside, but it also reflects your internal world. When you have piles of paper everywhere, heaps of clothes on the floor, a sink full of dishes, or an unmade bed it reflects your inner world—how you are feeling inside. Have you ever heard the saying, "Messy bed, messy head"? Well, there's a reason for it. When you take time to keep your personal space clean and clear of clutter, you can think with clarity. I often wash dishes or fold clothes just to relax. It's helpful to do things around the house that allow you to slow down, focus on one task at a time, and become more present. Pregnancy is another opportunity to slow down, and if you're a busy body this clearing period is a great way to start.

People can gather a lot about you simply by being in your home. Some areas are more fluid or comfortable; others are blocked and less functional. You can discover more about how to arrange your home in a way that reflects balance and stability by researching and incorporating the principles of feng shui, the ancient Chinese art form of aesthetics. But that's not what this book is about. Right now we're just doing a prepregnancy clean-out. So get out the heavy-duty garbage bags, call your local Goodwill, find your stoop-sale sign, and move some of that clutter out of your personal space. Open those closets and get rid of any clothing that doesn't make you feel and look amazing. The rule of thumb for wardrobe editing is very simple: "love it or leave it." If you are not in love with that dress that's been sitting in your closet for two years (because you *might* wear it) now's the time to leave it. Toss out those old worn-out shoes while you're at it.

Consider repainting your walls and rearranging your furniture. You are transforming your space into a royal queendom. Hang beautiful artwork. Bring natural elements indoors: buy some fresh herbs for window boxes, and if you can afford it, keep fresh-cut flowers in the house. Seashells are a nice touch because they symbolize fertility. I love chandeliers because they make the space feel elegant. When I wanted to invite love into my life I painted my living room a warm pink, put scented candles everywhere, and decorated with beautiful objects like crystals and pine cones to make my home a cozy place where I could envision myself with my future

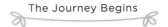

love. A good friend gave me a small fertility cow that I placed on my fireplace. You can bring in symbolic elements, too. Redesign your space so it inspires you. Then you will really enjoy spending time in your home, whether it's a 200-square-foot studio in NYC or a sprawling villa out on the prairie somewhere. Size doesn't matter when the space feels good.

Relationships: Toxic or Nurturing

When we take a good look at our lives, we must also look at our relationships. Some relationships are supportive, nourishing, and satisfying. But often, when we really take stock, we find we have a few toxic friendships in there, too—people who, no matter how much we may love them, are simply not positive influences. The key is to notice. It's not about cutting anyone off; it's about recognizing that you only have so much energy to spend. If you give your time to people who tire you, rather than people who inspire you, you are wasting the time you need to live the life of your dreams. Also, stress can change your cervical mucus pH and that affects fertility. We want to do our best to eliminate the stress we experience in relationships. We all have people in our lives who drain our energy—you know them because when you get off the phone with them you need to take a yoga class just to get back to feeling like yourself! That's what I call an energy vampire. News flash, mama: you're in total control of who you invite into your life on an intimate level. So take a look within and see if you have some energy vampires lurking around. If so, then change your behavior. Stop spending time with them, or reduce the amount of time you spend with them if you can't eliminate it altogether. If there are people in your family who tire you (which we all have to some degree) then the time is now—before you get pregnant—to negotiate healing those relationships. Use radical honesty and speak openly and truthfully about what is bothering you. I know it's a big thing to ask, but what many women find during pregnancy is that unresolved issues rise to the surface. This clearance period is a perfect time to address and clear up the past and do your best to let it go.

To get a sense of what relationships in your life may be toxic versus nourishing, answer the following questions:

- When I say no to this person do I feel bad?

- Do I often feel discouraged and drained when I speak to this person?

- Do I do things that don't feel good, like gossip, whine, and complain?

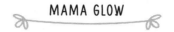

- Am I reluctant to share what's good in my life because it will upset the relationship?

- Do we have so much history together that I just don't feel right throwing it all away, even though there isn't much there?

If you said a big fat yes to more than three of these questions, then you are engaging in a toxic relationship. If you have several in your life, I encourage you to prioritize your self-care and focus on the healthy, loving relationships in your life. Now take a look at the following questions to gauge your healthy relationships:

- When I spend time with this person do I feel more like myself?

- Does this person understand me and is he or she a good listener?

- Am I a better person when we are together? Do I aspire to better things?

- Do I share my dreams and goals with this person because I know they care and want me to succeed?

- Is this person honest with me, and does the relationship make me grow?

If you answered yes to more than three of these questions, you are engaging in a nourishing relationship. Those are much easier to spot than the toxic ones. On a chemical level, when you surround yourself with loving relationships you counteract the stress response in your body, which I will talk more about later.

Sometimes a shift in your behavior can set the tone for change and correct a past hurt—rebuilding a stronger foundation. Before I conceived my son, my troubled relationship with my father reached its peak. We had not spoken in a few years. I felt righteous for excluding him from my life given his behavior during the four years leading up to the complete deterioration of our relationship. I was so angry. I knew that, with both of us being stubborn, the only way to find peace was to forgive my father. With the help of my son's father, I wrote a letter to my dad, apologizing and offering peace and forgiveness. I didn't know how the letter would be received, but I felt a huge relief. A few days later the phone rang and it was my father; we spoke for hours and laughed and cried. It was the beginning of a new relationship. The next time I saw him I shared the news that I was pregnant. I'm grateful I made this shift before my son was born so my father could participate in his life.

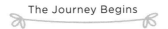

Who in your life is difficult—and how can you meet that person on a soul level, eye-to-eye, and find empathy? You can be in conscious dialogue without having to be right or make someone else wrong. When you start to forgive the people who you perceived as causing you harm, you end up freeing yourself. Forgiving doesn't mean condoning; it just means you are letting yourself off the hook emotionally. It's an incredible feeling to forgive. You no longer have to carry the emotional burden, which means the resentment, anger, and sadness no longer have a safe dwelling place in your physical body. Self-reflective practices, some of which I share in this book, will help you release some of the emotional blocks and glow full steam ahead.

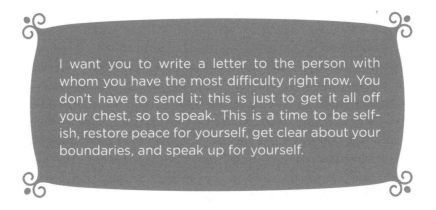

I want you to write a letter to the person with whom you have the most difficulty right now. You don't have to send it; this is just to get it all off your chest, so to speak. This is a time to be selfish, restore peace for yourself, get clear about your boundaries, and speak up for yourself.

Bag Lady

Whenever I travel, people are always amazed at how lightly I pack. No matter where I go, I carry my purse and just one bag, which fits neatly in the overhead compartment on an airplane. I don't see the logic in carrying so much that I become hindered and need to enlist help just to get to where I am going. Traveling through life is the same. You get to transition points where you have to stop and examine how much baggage you are carrying and make a decision if your bag exceeds the weight limit. You need to ask yourself, *What am I bringing with me?* and *What shall I leave behind?* Think about what baggage you've been carrying throughout your life, what emotions and thoughts have become associated with it, and why you haven't yet let it go. I have a lovely client who was in a new relationship and wanted to have a baby, yet she had this loathing for her ex-husband that was so strong it bled into other areas of her life. I had her complete the exercise

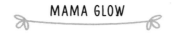
above, and we started to unpack this hatred that was weighing her down and affecting her new relationship.

Make sure the stuff you are carrying is worthy of toting around, honey. Take out your journal and write for five minutes. What baggage are you still carrying? If you can take only one bag with you, what's going inside?

Cleanse Your Limiting Beliefs

Part of the work of this book is to build your spiritual self-confidence, to help you become spiritually fit. That means I want you to tap into your groovy goddess, your inner diva, your soul power. But in order to harness that energy that lives within each of us, we have to get you out of your own way. Oftentimes it's our own beliefs about who we are and what we can and can't do, that keep us from realizing our full potential. I used to walk around playing this self-critical song over and over in my head like a Top 40 hit: *You're not worthy. You don't have anything important to say. You're not good enough.* Nodding your head? You find yourself playing that song over and over, too? Some of it comes from internalizing what other people have said to us. But most of it comes from being extremely judgmental of ourselves because of the culture we live in and what ideals we've been taught to buy into regarding beauty, gender, race, class, weight, hair texture, bust size, thigh circumference . . . the list goes on.

I'm not going to indulge your story—the thoughts that define your mental landscape about who you are. We all have a story, but these experiences don't have to define who we are, and they are not fuel for the glow. They prevent us from becoming our best selves. Positive, affirming thoughts are the fuel that propels us to a higher state of consciousness. This way of thinking takes us out of the framework of doubt and puts us in a positive framework of possibility. We start to see that, guess what, nobody fact-checked our limiting beliefs. We are telling ourselves unflattering, untrue stories, my friend. When we believe these stories they act as limitations, encouraging us to play small, which doesn't serve anyone. The good news is that we can choose to release the heavy thoughts and have a healthy inner dialogue with ourselves.

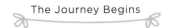

Take out your journal again and answer the following questions:

- What is my negative limiting soundtrack?

- How do I make myself small?

- What limiting beliefs do I have about myself?

Now, take a look at all you have written about yourself and decide what you are willing to release. Which of these limiting stories are you ready to let go of so you can move forward? What are you going to unpack and leave behind?

Now that we have begun to unpack our mental and emotional baggage, it's time to unpack our physical baggage, too.

Let the Janitor Do Her Job

Indulge me for a moment. Imagine your body as an office building, and your cleansing organs as the janitors. Just like any cleanup crew, your cleansing organs come in once the office building is closed for the day. In other words, our bodies do cellular repair and cleansing once we've wound down—during the times we are resting, or *supposed* to be resting. At an office building, what happens when someone decides to stay late and work? Why, the startled janitor says, "Pardon me! Sorry to bother you. I'll come back tomorrow." The janitor works only when the building is quiet; if you're partying in the building he'll just put off the work. After a while the garbage starts to overflow, papers start to pile up, dust gathers, rodents move in, and eventually the place has to be shut down for maintenance.

The same happens with the body. Your cleansing and repair organs can't do their job if you're hanging out until 1:30 A.M. every night, eating pizza, drinking, and partying. Instead of filtering clean blood back into the body, you're recirculating toxins through your bloodstream. Your internal cleansing organs (kidneys, liver, gallbladder, and colon) act as a filter for your blood. Like when a sponge gets full of water and the excess starts to drip out, when the organs are congested from toxic overload, excess contaminants spill out into the bloodstream. When our blood gets sludgy, we get sick. We look like we haven't slept. We just don't feel good. Problem is, some of us don't have an example of what feeling good even feels like, because our diet and habits have kept us on the fritz for so long.

One of my clients was an executive at a big financial institution, working ridiculous hours, entertaining over lavish meals, and traveling so much that her body could never catch up to the time zone she was in. Her body was so busy recovering from the lifestyle she was living that there was little time to devote to the baby she wanted to conceive. Once we made some pivotal lifestyle changes, including the adjustment of her work schedule, the addition of yoga four times per week, the elimination of meat and starchy foods, and the introduction of glow foods, her life shifted dramatically.

You want to have a baby, right? To do that, you want your body to work optimally. So don't lock out the cleanup crew, okay? Take this time to give your organs a break. Get seven to eight hours of sleep regularly. Allow yourself to enjoy the release and relief of letting go. Later in this section we will explore herbs to detoxify your system. And we'll focus on plant-based glow foods and juices to help clear the body and mind in preparation for the journey ahead.

The Womb-iverse

Now that you are releasing, you are making space for something new. You're cleaning up your relationships, arranging your living space, and cleansing yourself from within, all in preparation for a special guest who'll be making herself cozy for the next nine months or so. I say "or so," because your baby may turn out like mine and decide to stay an extra week. Who could blame him? The womb is the safest, most comfortable place to be. It's warm, dark, cozy, and rent-stabilized, with heat, water, and food included.

The womb is a sacred and magical space. It's the seat of creativity, where all of your dreams, aspirations, and goals are nourished in fertile soil and come to life. It's where life is spun into being, where spirit anchors itself to become flesh. This energy center is the very place that houses your glow, your divine inner light. There is an entire universe operating within your human body. I like to think of it as the "womb-iverse," and you can trust it.

You may have experienced difficulty conceiving in the past, including miscarriage and/or fertility issues. Now is the time to remember that you can create

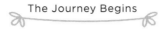
whatever you want to "womb-ifest" in your life. You can also begin to work with intention to prepare yourself for conceiving.

I have a client who is the mother of twins and has aspirations to become an accomplished writer but has never allowed herself to fully pursue her writing. She dreamed of having another baby but had a lot of trouble conceiving. It wasn't until she told me about all of her unborn dreams that we realized that she was blocking herself creatively on so many levels. One of my recommendations was for her to start writing every day, even if it was for leisure. She needed to stimulate her creative drive and take her dreams off the back burner. The writing seemed to make her more receptive; she started to feel more confident, which made her feel more sexy and happy in general. Eventually she did conceive and had a healthy baby boy.

This is the body that you will inhabit for the rest of your life! Learning to appreciate your own body can be a powerful tool for self-development. The word *midwife* is derived from the Anglo Saxon *med-wyf*, meaning "wise woman." If our ancestral midwives were here today, they'd emphasize the importance of providing clean ground where the embryo can take root and grow. Purification of the body through a diet of whole plant-foods and cleansing herbs can get your womb ready for action. Stay tuned, Chapter 2 will get us ready.

Weeding out the Wackness

A friend once called me to personally give me his new phone number. I asked him why he was going through such an effort to change a number that he'd had for ages, and he said, "I'm just weeding out the wackness, clearing out my social garden so all that's left are flowers." I loved this, and the same idea goes for getting ready to conceive. Clearing out the weeds is an important step in preparing ourselves for the baby we dream about.

When I talk about clearing things out, I am referring to clearing out harmful substances, wack relationships, and bad habits. But I'm also talking about using real-life weeds (affectionately known as herbs) to clear blockages in the body. Weeds are often misunderstood because most of us don't know what to do with them. They proliferate in our gardens, outgrow the grass . . . they are everywhere, even growing from the cracks in the sidewalks. How could something growing from the sidewalk be good for you, you wonder? Well, think of them as Mother Nature's first line of defense. What if I told you that the weeds I'm talking about can be powerful blood builders, can restore hormonal balance, and can tonify some of the major organs of the female reproductive system? (Maybe you'd think twice before trampling them or letting your dog pee on them!)

The use of medicinal herbs to heal and maintain balance in the body is common to all indigenous cultures. I am a big believer in the power of herbs, so part of your Mama Glow cleansing regimen includes the use of these pixie plants. Dandelion and burdock root are cleansing bitter herbs that have an astringent effect on the liver. The liver serves a vital function in almost every system in your body, from hormone and digestive enzyme production to blood filtration. In traditional Chinese medicine, the liver is the organ associated with anger. So it's good to keep in mind that when you start purging your system, your emotions may be unsettled. I have spoken to clients who say that by day three of their detox they feel angry. A willingness to sort through your unresolved feelings as you undergo this cleansing process is key to removing emotional blocks, too.

In the prepregnancy detox that follows, I recommend balancing herbs that specifically tone the reproductive system (including yarrow, raspberry leaves, and lady's mantle) and those that balance hormonal functions (such as chasteberry and false unicorn root). These will clear and fortify the womb and promote fertility. The herbal tinctures can be taken in water or tea by the dropper. You can also take these herbs as teas, which can be purchased online at Mountain Rose Herbs (MountainRoseHerbs.com) or Frontier Co-op (FrontierCoop.com), or at your local apothecary. There are several brands of commercial bagged teas you can try if loose teas aren't an option, including Traditional Medicinals, Celebration Herbals, and Yogi Tea.

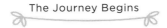

Fertili-Tea (4 servings)

Try this recipe for uterine tone and general reproductive health. Drink a cup daily (this can replace a morning coffee ritual).

1 tablespoon chasteberry
1 tablespoon peppermint
1 tablespoon red raspberry leaf
1 tablespoon white tea
1 tablespoon lady's mantle
1 tablespoon nettle leaf
Raw agave nectar or honey, to taste
    (optional)

Mix loose herbs in a teapot or tea infuser. Add 1 quart of boiling water and steep for 5 minutes. Can be served hot or chilled. Sweeten, if desired.

We're well under way and ready to get your diet on track—and full of glow foods. In the next chapter you'll learn about the detox plan and how to cleanse your way to the best pregnancy you could imagine!

CHAPTER 2

IN THE KITCHEN

Intro to the Glow Plan

I went vegetarian when I was 12 years old. It wasn't for any philosophical reason at first. I wanted to be like my babysitter, Danielle, who was a wonderful role model and happened to be vegetarian at the time. I didn't grow up eating much meat, so the transition was seamless and I never once looked back. Over the years I studied food a great deal and learned a lot about how my body responds to certain foods. I feel my very best on a vegan diet with lots of raw foods in the summertime and green juice year-round. This is a diet I maintained throughout my pregnancy and one that my son embraces as well. I consider this not only good nutrition, but powerful medicine, too.

The medicinal value of food has been acknowledged for thousands of years. In recent times scientific research has shown hundreds of beneficial nutrients in the foods that we eat. Knowing about these nutrients and how they work in our diet helps us boost our immune systems, nourish ourselves and our babies, and protect ourselves against ailments. *Before* you begin your pregnancy journey is the best time to explore glow foods—super-foods packed with antioxidants, minerals, and powerful nutrients that are particularly effective in boosting the body's natural defenses, promoting optimal wellness, and activating the glow. Some of these glow foods include beets, kale, grapefruit, blueberries, quinoa, avocado, almonds, Brazil nuts, shitake mushrooms, sweet potatoes, goji berries, hempseeds, acai, tempeh, and garlic.

Glow foods are rich in nutrients, and are easy to digest and assimilate. They don't cause wacky cravings, constipation, or indigestion, and they are absorbed slowly by the body, keeping insulin levels low. Glow foods promote optimal circulation of oxygen and nutrients to cells and promote healthy weight maintenance. And if you're wondering about your skin, nails, and hair, you can be sure that they, too, will shimmer. (I don't call them glow foods for nothin'!)

Plant foods are balanced, abundant in vitamins, minerals, antioxidants, and phytochemicals. They bind with toxins in your tissues and help pass impurities out of the body, leaving you luminous. Just like we have blood, plants have chlorophyll. Liquid chlorophyll is helpful to our bodies, balancing blood sugar levels and acting as a blood builder, carrying vitamins and minerals into the cells and oxygenating and fortifying the blood.

When your body is in a state of balance, you are more likely to make choices that sustain health and vitality. You are more likely to put *you* first, because you already feel good and want to maintain that feeling. You don't need me to remind you what it feels like when you are out of balance. You make food and behavior choices that have harsh effects. This might mean skipping your workouts for a week because of stress or eating fast food or takeout and a pack of Twizzlers a day.

Glow foods help manage cravings, while bringing your body into balance, because you are eating natural whole foods—rather than overly processed foods.

Eating a diet full of glow foods means you are eating in step with nature. Eat locally and you get extra credit, my friend. Nature gives us the foods we need each season to prepare us for what lies ahead during that season. In the spring we get foods that are cleansing and regenerative—like leafy greens, lemon, and onion. In the summer we get foods that are hydrating and cooling—watermelon, cucumber, and berries, to name a few. In the fall we indulge in seasonal foods that ground us and help prepare our bodies for the cooler months ahead. Think beets, soft squashes, and legumes. Finally, in the winter we have hard squashes, hearty greens, and grains to keep us warm until the sun comes back!

Glow foods protect us from health issues, too. I'm a big fan of the cruciferous crusaders like broccoli, kale, collards, mustard greens, and watercress. They contain a substance that inhibits estrogen that cause tumors in the breast tissue, protecting the breasts from cysts and cancer. Fiber is also good for limiting estrogen, as it binds with the hormone and moves it out of the body. The more fiber you eat, the better. Vegetarian women eliminate two to three times more estrogen

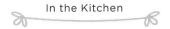

than their nonveggie counterparts. (Fiber also reduces PMS symptoms, ladies . . . I'm just saying.)

Oxidants—also known as free radicals—are highly reactive oxygen molecules that cause the breakdown of proteins and enzymes that make up our cells. Oxidants occur as a normal part of body functions including metabolism and digestion, but when they are rampant in the system they can cause problems. Oxidants cause skin dehydration and wrinkle formation as well as a host of degenerative diseases. The primary lifestyle causes of oxidant overload include stress, smoking (including secondhand smoke), dietary fat, X-rays, processed foods, industrial toxins, chemical food additives, and too much ultraviolet sunlight. (As much as I love hanging out in the sun, I suggest limiting exposure to protect your skin.) So what's the solution for oxidants in your system? You guessed it, antioxidants! The major power players include vitamins C, E, and B6, beta-carotene, selenium, magnesium, glutathione—all of which can be found in glow foods.

Time to Get Down to Business: Cleansing for Pregnancy

Now that you know a little more about what glow foods can do for you, it's time for a concrete prescription. The following guidelines will first help you get to the place where you are releasing the old buildup from your system—letting it all go. Then they'll start to build your body back up for glow time: your pregnancy! Remember your baby is made up of what you eat now, not just what you eat during pregnancy. Your body will pull nutrients from your tissues to develop your baby.

Healthy detox components include the following: colon cleansing, moderate exercise, relaxation, meditation, cleaning out your home, organizing your life, spending time in nature, experiencing therapeutic touch, and processing and healing personal issues. Start doing things today that will matter tomorrow. Don't put off your quest. You'll never have more time than you do right now. You owe it to yourself. Let's go! Follow these recommendations to get lean, mean, clean, and ready for your baby.

Glow Guideline #1: Stay Fluid

Our bodies are 70 to 75 percent water. And our brains are *85 percent* water! It is water that energizes and activates the solid matter—our bones, muscles, connective tissue, and so on. If you don't drink enough water, some functions of the

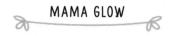
body will suffer. Dehydration produces system disturbances. A well-hydrated body will ensure better digestion, increased assimilation of nutrients, and a robust metabolism. You also need adequate water to produce reproductive fluids. Glow foods like fresh fruits and veggies contain lots of water and help you stay hydrated. Watermelon, celery, and cucumbers are a great way to get more water in your system. Coconut water, a glow food, qualifies as an excellent tonic for hydration, electrolytes, and trace minerals that come directly from the sea, and it's reputed to increase libido. Your pregnancy will require extra fluid so why not get in the habit of drinking well now?

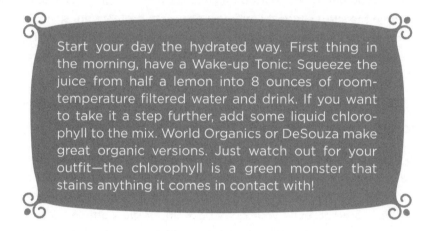

Start your day the hydrated way. First thing in the morning, have a Wake-up Tonic: Squeeze the juice from half a lemon into 8 ounces of room-temperature filtered water and drink. If you want to take it a step further, add some liquid chlorophyll to the mix. World Organics or DeSouza make great organic versions. Just watch out for your outfit—the chlorophyll is a green monster that stains anything it comes in contact with!

Glow Guideline #2: Get Up and Go!

Really now, by this point do I need to tell you that you should be exercising? It's not up for debate. You *do* have time for it, so no excuses. You make time for everything else you want to do, so choose to make exercise a priority by picking something that you actually *enjoy doing*. Then do it—in the mornings whenever possible. When you work out at the start of your day it decreases your appetite and stimulates the thyroid to burn calories all day long. This is especially important if you are looking to drop a few pounds prior to getting pregnant. And here's a bonus, you may increase your libido just by working out!

Some favorite morning activities of mine are yoga, walking, jogging, swimming, and spinning. Add some resistance training at the end of the workout to further stimulate the fat-burning process. This might include push-ups, pull-ups, crunches, or squats. When it's warmer outside our bodies naturally desire more

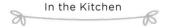

sunlight and activity, so rev it up during the warm months, hot stuff! When it's cooler outside you can move more gently to protect joints and muscles. Carve out some time in your busy schedule to do some of the things you love to do outdoors. Rollerblading, bike riding, recreational sports, dancing, walking—whatever it is you enjoy doing. When you do what you love, you're happiest, and you'll be able to exercise without effort.

Glow Guideline #3: Eat Your Veggies!

I've adopted the slogan "Eat your veggies!" from my diva sister Kris Carr, who manages her cancer through diet and lifestyle. If you're looking for a place to start, think green. Green juice and green foods are anti-inflammatory, antiseptic, and anticancer, and they've loaded with digestive enzymes and trace minerals. Plus they destroy toxins. I like to say that when you're green inside, you're clean in-side. Greens are loaded with folate, which every woman should have in her diet if she plans on getting pregnant. We'll learn more about folate in the next section. We need it most in the first weeks of pregnancy to ensure proper development of the baby's skeletal and nervous system. So start by filling up on upward-reaching leafy greens: kale, collards, arugula, mizuna, and so on. Few of us eat the minimum USDA recommended three cups of leafy greens *per week*. It shouldn't be so hard! Calorie for calorie, dark green leafy vegetables contain perhaps the most concen-trated source of nutrition of any food. They are rich sources of minerals (including iron, calcium, potassium, and magnesium) and vitamins, including vitamins K, C, E, and many of the B varieties. They also provide phytonutrients, which protect our cells from damage. Dark green leaves even contain small amounts of omega-3 fats, which are helpful for maternal health and fetal development, including the cardiac and central nervous systems. Greens help to regulate blood sugar, break down fats, and alkalize the blood. Moreover, eating lower on the food chain (i.e., eating more vegetables than animal proteins) can help prevent the consumption of many environmental toxins that are more concentrated in animal foods. Those toxins find their way into our liver and fat cells.

All of our energy comes from the sun. We get it from plants, or animals that have eaten plants. Why not just go right to the source? You can't go wrong with powerful greens like lamb's quarters, watercress, purslane, mesclun, mustard, tur-nips, kale, dandelion, and collards. (Spicy greens like arugula and mizuna work well with tangy dressings.)

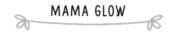

Really, I could go on and on here. But I'm done with my PSA. Here's your prescription: Gobble two salads a day and down a green juice in the morning. (Oh, and make kale your new BFF. Okay?)

Glow Guideline #4: Get Your Sea On!

Minerals compose the complex matrix of the human body and salt is one of those vital minerals. We need salt for protein digestion, adrenal function, brain development, and cellular regeneration. But in excess, salt attracts moisture—meaning you get swelling and dampness in the body. Here's the good news: you can get the sodium your body needs without the ill effects of salt by eating yummy sea vegetables. Sea vegetables, which contain organic sodium bound in carbon, make it easy to eliminate carbon dioxide from the body and are a goldmine of power-packed nutrition.

Table salt (the iodized white stuff) weakens immunity, increases blood pressure, can cause edema, and contributes to weight gain. Sea vegetables, on the other hand, contain all 56 minerals and trace elements required for your body's physiological functions. They strengthen immunity and can even reverse high blood pressure and edema. I like to use dulse flakes and sprinkle them over my food. I also take kombu and other seaweeds and add them to my stews or beans for flavor and minerals. My son loves nori strips—the seaweed used to wrap sushi—with a little avocado, hummus, and cucumber.

If you're using regular salt, choose gray-, pink-, or beige-colored varieties—the coloration indicates the presence of minerals. The ocean contains all minerals that exist; ocean water heals us. Seawater is Mother Earth's cellular fluid. Spending time in the ocean is good for you, especially while cleansing. The salt or saline content of amniotic fluid is the same as that of the oceans. See how connected we are to nature? The rule of thumb when it comes to sea vegetables and pregnancy is that any plant growing in the ocean can help grow a healthy baby.

Glow Guideline #5: Soak It Out

Yes, you have to run a bath for this guideline. If you aren't near a decent body of seawater, the bathtub is your best bet for getting minerals through your skin. It is quite nice to soak. It helps to relax your nervous system and calm your brain waves, which is important as you prepare to conceive. Try a mixture of epsom

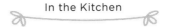

salts, dead sea salts, essential oils, and hot water. It's the perfect solution to a long day. To really do it big—glow-girl style—treat yourself to a nice scented candle or two, shut off the phone and the light, and relax in the tub for a minimum of 15 minutes. Commit to doing this a few times a week to relax the body and ease the mind. You and your baby-to-be will thank you!

Glow Guideline #6: Got Fat?

Fats and oils are not evil, ladies. In fact, they are necessary for a healthy pregnancy. I'm going to help you choose the right ones. Most processed oils are loaded with free radicals. High temperature processing causes the weak carbon bonds of the unsaturated fatty acids to break apart (especially omega-3 fatty acid), thereby creating dangerous free radicals. This means processed oils are damaging to the reproductive organs and can cause premature wrinkling. The process of refining takes out the essence of the oil, so it no longer contains chlorophyll, lecithin, or minerals. Eating these oils robs the body of nutrients and contributes to cell mutation. Once heated, the oils become unstable. So steer clear of margarine and spreads, as most are made from rancid expeller-pressed oils. They are partially hydrogenated fats, the polite term for trans fats. Instead eat cold-pressed oils like olive oil, used as a finishing oil—don't cook it at high heat. Cold-pressed oils are pressed with an oil-stone at room temperature. If you have expeller-pressed or refined oils in the cabinets, get rid of them.

Your prepregnancy is also time to load up on omega-3 sources: flaxseeds, hempseeds, chia seeds and oils, leafy greens, walnuts, and pumpkin seeds. You need omegas to produce sexual fluids, and for ovum production. Sterility is more common when there is low omega-3 production. There is an abundance of these oils in everything that grows in the plant and animal kingdoms, but especially in cold-climate crops like mustard greens, kale, beets, and collards.

If fats are such a tricky terrain to navigate, why not cut them out altogether? Simple: a fat-free diet is not going to make it easy to get pregnant. Not to mention what it will (and won't) do for fetal growth, the vascular system, and proper brain development. You need your omegas! So get on the ball, girlfriend. Women without regular menstrual periods should especially look to add in more oils and higher-quality calories. (And reduce stress on mind and body, just saying.)

Unrefined oils are cold-pressed without exposure to heat. Try extra-virgin olive oil, hempseed oil, and flaxseed oils to finish off a great salad. Adding oil to salads is an easy way to get good-quality fats. You deserve full-fat salad dressing, so stop

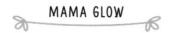
reaching for the fat-free one on the salad bar. When you put your salad together, add a little avocado and tomato to get that lycopene and vitamin A. And don't forget to add a tablespoon of flax, borage, or evening primrose oil to your morning smoothie!

Glow Guideline #7: Soy Is Your Frenemy

You think it's your friend, but guess what . . . it's not. There was a soy product craze in the '90s and nearly everyone jumped on the bandwagon. We were all sipping our soy lattes, nibbling on our soy nuts, and scarfing our tofu sandwiches thinking we were being super-healthy eaters. What we didn't know was that we were actually contributing to some possible health concerns down the line. Soy may be good for heart health, prevention of some cancers, and healthy bones, but it has also been linked to allergies, thyroid issues, and negative effects on reproductive health. When it comes to pregnancy, soy can be problematic because its estrogens may interfere with fertility. In fact, when you are cleansing the body for pregnancy, it's best to stay away from any foods that can cause allergens—including the Sensitive 7: soy, wheat, dairy, eggs, peanuts, sugar, and corn.

Soy contains toxins. Its phytic acid blocks absorption of calcium, magnesium, and zinc. Protease inhibitors are a class of proteins that block proper digestion, and soybeans are rich in protease inhibitors. Soy's isoflavones—plant estrogens—can cause thyroid problems, digestive disorders, and headaches. You don't have to get rid of soy completely, but dump the worst soy-related products. These include soymilk, which is highly processed, and textured soy protein—the fake meat you find in the frozen food section. The only versions of soy that are really okay during pregnancy are tempeh, which is fermented soy, and organic soybeans (edamame). Keep quantities limited to three ounces per serving, and don't eat them every day.

Glow Guideline #8: Super-Food Me!

You've heard of super-foods, but did you know that many of the popular super-foods on the market today are also glow foods? When properly incorporated into your diet, these super-foods can do wonders for your overall wellness. Here are just a few:

- Spirulina, or blue-green algae, is 63 percent protein—the highest planetary source of protein. It also contains vitamin A, nucleic acids,

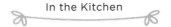

chlorophyll, and iron, and cleanses the body as it builds it—a terrific addition to your detox!

- Cacao is the strongest antioxidant on earth; it relaxes muscles and builds strong bones and teeth. It contains more magnesium than any other food, helping to balance brain chemistry, regulate blood pressure, and keep bowels regular. By increasing neurotransmitters in our brains, cacao promotes a feeling of rejuvenation, positive outlook, and a sense of well-being—it's nature's antidepressant.

- Macá invigorates the endocrine system, balancing hormones. It increases stamina, combats acne and PMS symptoms, and increases libido in both men and women. It contains vitamin B12, protein, loads of calcium, and all of the essential amino acids.

- Goji berry is a powerful antioxidant, contains 21 trace minerals, and is a complete protein source. It increases human growth hormone, reversing some of the effects of aging. Benefits include improved eyesight, restoration of hair color, increased libido, and enhanced mood.

- Hempseeds are a complete protein source and have sulfur-bearing amino acids, helping to build strong nails and hair, and promoting beautiful skin. Hempseeds detoxify the liver and support a healthy pancreas. They rejuvenate connective tissue and contain 21 trace minerals.

Talk about bathing yourself from inside out! These powerful glow foods are cleansing, fortifying, and boast off-the-charts nutrition profiles. My favorite way to get these in my system is to whip them into a smoothie—but you can eat them however you like. Just eat them!

Glow Guideline #9: Cut the Crap

By now, you are probably already making changes to support your health—including cutting out some foods that are, nutritionally speaking, total fluff. You're probably ready to dive right in and make lasting changes, too. If you have processed foods like chips, cakes, and cookies sitting around for "just in case," kindly collect them and toss them. Yes, put the book down right now, walk to the kitchen, and collect at least three things that you can live without. Liberate yourself.

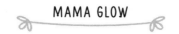
Processed foods increase weight and blood lipids (trigylcerides), and 20 percent of the triglycerides you ingest become blood cholesterol. Find healthy alternatives to satisfy your munchies. For instance, if you're a nacho chip lover try carrot sticks and hummus or flax crackers with veggie pâté. Try kale chips instead of potato chips, or dip some apple slices in almond butter.

Glow Guideline #10: Call It Quits with Caffeine

Caffeine is found in coffee, some teas, cola drinks, and, of course, our beloved chocolate. Caffeine is addictive, making it one of the world's most widely used legal drugs. It can cause a number of health concerns, including interference with iron absorption, increased heart rate and blood pressure, stomach irritation, and headaches. Excess caffeine in pregnancy has been linked with low birth weight in babies. There are lots of alternatives to that cup of joe that will make you feel more at ease with this recommendation. Try Teeccino (an herbal coffee alternative), yerba mate, licorice tea, rooibos tea, and on the cooler side, an acai smoothie—which you will find in the recipes section in Appendix B. Wean yourself by decreasing your daily intake by half to start, then whittle it down until the habit is broken.

Glow Guideline #11: Know Your ABCs

A multivitamin is your first line of defense during pregnancy, protecting you from illness, boosting your immunity, and growing your baby. Here's a prepregnancy vitamin primer:

- Vitamins A, C, E, and selenium are powerful antioxidants. As with all vitamins, taking these with food will help you absorb them rather than flush them right out.

- Folic acid is a B-complex vitamin needed by the body to manufacture red blood cells. A deficiency of this vitamin causes certain types of anemia. Folic acid is extremely important during pregnancy, aiding in baby's brain development. All women in childbearing years should take it.

- Vitamin C by itself is best taken in food rather than as a supplement. This is important during pregnancy, because too much vitamin C in supplement form can cause preterm labor. It's water-soluble, meaning it isn't stored in the body and needs to be replaced daily.

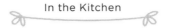

Here's a vitamin-rich glow tip: Don't take all of your supplements at once. Minerals should be taken at night for tissue repair and cellular rejuvenation. Vitamins should be taken in the morning. Also, choose brands that are food-based. They remind the body of a food source. That said, there isn't a replacement for a healthy diet of glow foods—so cutting corners and taking supplements instead of eating fresh whole foods is not the way to go about this program. For example, vitamin C is 250 times more active in whole, fresh foods than in a pill form. In other words, there's something to be said for eating the real deal.

Just because you're in the health food store doesn't mean everything you see is good for you. You still have to read the labels and make sure you aren't being tricked into getting something unhealthy just because it reads "all natural." At the other end of the spectrum, some of us are willing to spend more money on our wardrobe than we are on our food. We'll buy the hottest handbag or designer stiletto and pay top dollar for it, but when it comes to our food choices we aren't picking the best quality every time. Why wouldn't you care just as much about what's going *into* your body as what you wear *on* it? It's expensive to eat cheap foods—they cost a lot down the line in terms of your health. You can pay now or pay later, my dear. When you shift your perception of food to one where food is on your side—where it's your partner in manifesting a healthy relationship with your body—you will be inspired to make choices that support your overall well-being.

Kick the Dairy Dose

You are about to produce your own milk, so you should already be weaned! Many of the reproductive issues I see in my clients stem from an overconsumption of milk products. This is a silent source of illness in Western culture. Once you drink that good ole glass of milk, the seemingly harmless lactose is transformed into galactose. Your body responds to galactose—a potent form of sugar—by producing enzymes that metabolize the sugar. When you have excess galactose in your system from too many dairy products, your body's ability to get rid of it quickly is inhibited. This has an adverse effect on the female reproductive system. Beyond pregnancy issues, including infertility, galactose has been linked to ovarian cancer—which, if you ask me, is enough reason to give up the cookies and milk.

Proteins in cow's milk have been linked to a number of ailments, including asthma, digestive issues, chronic mucus, runny nose, earaches, and eczema. Milk blocks iron absorption, too. Without adequate iron, the body can't make hemoglobin (whose job is to carry oxygen in the blood). So another possible outcome of the dairy habit is anemia, which produces fatigue. Lord knows, as a pregnant woman you don't need anything else to make you feel tired.

Drinking cow's milk also causes a rapid increase in insulinlike growth factor (IGF-1), high levels of which have been linked to breast and prostate cancers. Many nonorganic milk products are laced with antibiotics, recombinant bovine growth hormone, and pesticides from the feed. Pesticides concentrate in the cow's fat cells—and of course, are transferred into the milk.

Research shows that contrary to conventional understanding, dairy products actually put you at *risk* for osteoporosis. High levels of protein in milk promote the loss of calcium through the kidneys. So don't believe them when they say you need to drink milk or eat yogurt for calcium. Your best bet for calcium is . . . drumroll please . . . leafy green veggies! The only reason milk has calcium to begin with is because cows eat grass. Nowadays our bovine buddies are packed into industrial farms eating grain—which does not contain calcium, and which they aren't designed to eat. So when the milk goes for processing it has to be enriched with the nutrients that naturally occur in a grass-fed diet—including vitamin D and other minerals.

Vitamin D lowers the risk of cancer and bone fractures, but guess what—you don't need to get it from enriched dairy. In fact, there is no way to get vitamin D from natural foods (with the exception of a teensy bit you can get from fish). The premier way to get your D fix is through sunshine. Your body produces vitamin D when you are exposed to sunlight, UVB rays. You need up to 30 minutes exposure on your face, arms, and legs twice per week. Take a nice walk in the sun in the mornings between 7 and 9 A.M. to get the best quality of light without the harmful UVA rays. Go without sunglasses to maximize the vitamin D intake, since the light has to hit your retina for vitamin D to be synthesized. To absorb the sunlight, it also helps to wear fewer layers. If you're not a sun worshiper, then try vitamin D drops, which you can purchase online; Nature's Answer makes a great vitamin D-3 liquid formula that I recommend.

The long and short of it is that dairy is not an essential part of the human diet. If you are struggling with this concept, consider that most cultures of the world are dairy free. In fact, many populations are lactose intolerant. It's interesting that in developing countries around the globe we see a higher incidence of breastfeeding and for longer periods of time. Yet when those children wean from the breast, they do not go to other species' milk for supplementation. Mother Nature in her genius design would never have crafted human babies to be dependent upon the milk of cows for survival. In our culture, where many of us haven't been nursed at the breast and haven't had that intimate connection with our mother, it's no wonder we comfort ourselves with dairy foods.

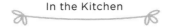

It gets even easier to understand when we learn that there are small amounts of morphine in cow's milk. Known as *casomorphins,* these opiates form as casein (milk) when digested. Dr. Neal Barnard of the Physicians Committee for Responsible Medicine is quoted in an article from the National Health Association as saying, "Casein, the fundamental protein in cow's milk, breaks apart in the digestive process to release chemicals called casomorphins, and the casomorphins are casein-derived, morphine-like substances." Cheese contains loads of casomorphins. Dr. Barnard says, "It is the process of cheese-making, when all the liquid is pressed together, which leaves just pure casein and fat. And it's the purest form of the casein—and once in your digestive track it breaks down into casomorphins." So cheese is essentially dairy crack! You can't help eating it because it is addictive.

So why do so many of us feel so bad after eating milk and cheese products? It may have to do with lactose (milk sugar). About 30 to 50 million Americans have problems digesting lactose, which can result in some pretty nasty side effects—think gas, bloating, cramps, diarrhea, and even extremes like nausea and vomiting.

Want to avoid a lactose overdose in the future? Cut out the dairy, my friend. It's worth it. I don't like taking things away from people, but dairy is something we know is just not necessary for our health and, in fact, hinders our well-being.

So what are my cheese-addicted and milk-fiend friends to do? There's hope. Here are some tasty alternatives to milk and cheese:

- Try dairy-free cheese. There are some "cheeses" on the market that don't contain any cheese at all. Try brands like Daiya Foods and Galaxy Nutritional Foods for cheese alternatives from cream cheese to cheddar. Some vegan varieties even melt when heated! If you are not as fond of soy-based cheeses (and I'm not a fan myself), how about a nut cheese? A brand I love is Dr. Cow Tree Nut Cheese. It comes in a variety of flavors and the texture is like that of cream cheese. Plus it's enzyme-rich because it's cultured.

- Try nut milk. Most people know about soymilk as an alternative to cow's milk, but why not try almond milk, hemp milk, or cashew milk? There are ready-made varieties available at your local health food store. It is also very easy to make your own version at home.

  There are lots of commercial brands out there that you can buy, but once you start making your own nut milk, there is no turning back. It's easy, better tasting, and better for you. Try the basic almond milk recipe on the next page. This can serve as a base for your smoothies, baked goods, or morning granola.

Basic Almond Milk (6 servings)

2 cups almonds, soaked
7 cups purified water
2 to 3 pitted dates or 2 to 3 tablespoons
    raw agave nectar
2 to 3 drops of natural vanilla extract
    (optional)

Soak almonds in a bowl with 4 cups of water for a minimum of 3 hours. Then rinse. Place almonds and 3 cups of water in a blender and process at the highest speed. Strain mixture into a bowl through a fine sieve, nut milk bag, or a couple of layers of cheesecloth. Rinse blender and return the strained liquid to blender. Add dates or agave nectar and vanilla extract, if using, and blend again. This milk will keep five days tightly sealed in the refrigerator.

You can substitute different nuts here in lieu of almonds. Try cashews or Brazil nuts. (I used Brazil nut milk to wean my son off my breast milk; see page 240 for the recipe.) Even hempseeds can be used. There is no need to soak prior to blending and no need to strain. Hemp offers a pleasant but strong aftertaste, so make sure to flavor it according to your preference. In the recipes section (Appendix B), you'll find recipes for all of these variations.

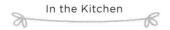

The Glow Prepregnancy Detox Plan

Now that you're following your guidelines, it's time to put them together into a detox plan. This simple plan can be used for a finite amount of time as a detox, but my suggestion is to begin to incorporate the elements of the detox into your maintenance diet as well. A little green goes a long way!

People get excited for their detox programs—buying their kits with pills and shakes, gearing up for their juice cleanses. These programs often have us soaring sky high, feeling great for a few days—only to *re-tox* a few days after breaking our fast. This glow plan is different. It's gentle and not at all difficult to maintain. When we get involved in fasts, especially for the first time, the experience can be intense. People often harbor a sense of failure if they haven't been realistic, setting the bar too high.

Not so with the glow. My prepregnancy plan is divided into three levels that correspond with where you are lifestyle-wise: Glitz, Glimmer, and Glow. My recommendation is that you work with the plan for a minimum of 7 days, but the full effect is easier to see over a longer period like 21 days. If you were to do each level for a week, that would ease you into the detox and put you at 21 days—but follow whatever combination works for you. You may just want to do the Glitz level for 21 days and not try the other levels. That would be fine—do what feels right for your body. Approach every day as fresh and new, and focus only on the day that lies before you. If it feels good, continue with it the next day. Keep operating one day at a time, and before you know it you'll be at your goal. You will need a juicer and a blender—preferably a high-speed blender like Blendtec or Vitamix—for the juice preparation. For all three programs it's advised that you exercise. My recommendation is yoga because it's a gentle way to stimulate the organs while also getting in some strength and flexibility training.

Level I: The Glitz

If you have never cleansed or fasted before, the Glitz detox is perfect for you. It's very basic and is all about replacing problem foods with plant-based foods and smoothies. If you are using dairy, soy, caffeine, and sugar, the Glitz is the first step toward clearing out the nutritional clutter. Those substances really interfere with your ability to get your shine on. This cleansing yet balancing approach will set you on your way.

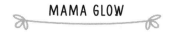

Glitz Detox Program

- *What's In:* Whole grains, legumes, nuts, seeds, raw or steamed veggies, fruits (low-glycemic), and smoothies.

- *What's Out:* Animal products, dairy, gluten, caffeine, alcohol, processed grains, and refined sugar.

- *What You Can Expect:* Reduced cravings, increase of nutrients readily available in your body, and an increase in energy.

Plant foods contain water and fiber, and are low in calories, which make them perfect for your detox plan. You will want to stock up your kitchen with whole foods so you're prepared for the next 7 to 21 days of transition. In terms of portions, I leave that up to you. The key is to remove processed food from the diet. This allows the liver to detoxify, giving a nice sheen to your complexion.

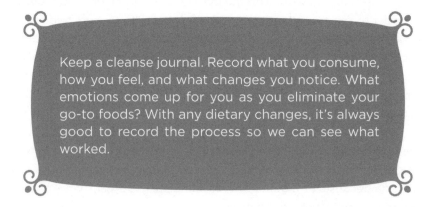

Keep a cleanse journal. Record what you consume, how you feel, and what changes you notice. What emotions come up for you as you eliminate your go-to foods? With any dietary changes, it's always good to record the process so we can see what worked.

Breakfast: Drink a glass of room-temperature filtered water with the juice of half a lemon to balance pH, aid in digestion, and boost your immune system. Do this as soon as you wake up so that you can allow at least 20 minutes before you eat. For breakfast you can choose something soothing like quinoa porridge, a grapefruit, an acai and blueberry smoothie, or granola with almond milk.

Lunch: Three quarters of your plate should be covered in salad greens and other raw veggies. The remainder can be steamed veggies, beans, or soup.

Snack: Something light that is no larger than the palm of your hand. A piece of fruit, a handful of almonds, or flax crackers with hummus.

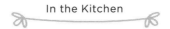

Dinner: This is a no-brainer, and similar to what you had for lunch. Seventy-five percent of your meal should be raw mixed greens with a tasty dressing (try my Goddess Herb Dressing recipe on page 82), then the remaining 25 percent should be a grain or legume—like quinoa tabbouleh or lentil salad with sliced avocado on the side.

Drink adequate filtered water in between meals, which will help the elimination process.

Glitz Detox Sample Day

Upon Rising: 10 ounces warm water with the juice of half a lemon
Breakfast: Rockstar Granola (page 236) with Basic Almond Milk (page 28) and blueberries
Lunch: Mixed green salad with Lemon Tahini Dressing (page 275)
Snack: Cucumber, carrots, and hummus
Dinner: Steamed veggies, black beans, and brown rice

Level II: The Glimmer

This plan adds raw food to the mix. This program is for people who want to take it a step further and incorporate green juice, which I think of as "liquid glow." For the Glimmer program you will need a juicer or access to fresh, pressed juices. The rule for green juice is that for every fruit you must include two veggies. For instance: you could have a juice with apple, pineapple, kale, cucumber, celery, parsley, and ginger. The Glimmer program also allows for steamed veggies, hearty salads, and smoothies.

Glimmer Detox Program

- *What's In:* Quinoa, nuts, seeds, raw or steamed veggies, fruits (low glycemic), and smoothies. Strive for fewer fruits and more vegetables.

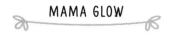

- *What's Out:* Animal products, dairy, gluten, caffeine, alcohol, processed grains, refined sugar, and all grains except quinoa, which is a complete protein and gluten free.

- *What You Can Expect:* Mental clarity, frequent urination due to toxin elimination, decrease in constipation, bright skin and clear eyes, and increased energy.

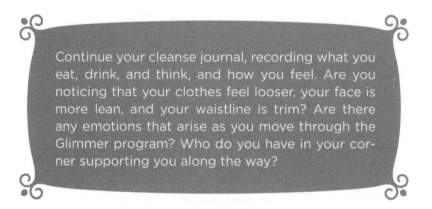

Continue your cleanse journal, recording what you eat, drink, and think, and how you feel. Are you noticing that your clothes feel looser, your face is more lean, and your waistline is trim? Are there any emotions that arise as you move through the Glimmer program? Who do you have in your corner supporting you along the way?

Breakfast: Again, we greet the day with a glass of room-temperature filtered water with the juice of half a lemon. Breakfast options include green juice, smoothie, fresh berries, or grapefruit.

Lunch: Three-quarters of your plate will feature salad greens with veggies. Steamed veggies could include: broccoli, zucchini, cauliflower, carrots, or squash. The small portion of your plate is reserved for a mild grain like quinoa, and beans like garbanzo, black, or kidney beans. Color balance is important here; try to include a variety of different colors on your plate.

Snack: When snacking on nuts and seeds limit consumption to 3 ounces: sunflower seeds, raw almonds, and Brazil nuts. Instead of eating your snack, you can drink it. Try an 8-ounce green juice or smoothie like Goji Sunset (see page 257) to give you that energy boost you may need to get through the rest of your busy day.

Dinner: Steamed greens and squash on 75 percent of your plate. Flavor your veggies with an oil-based dressing to ensure you get your fat-soluble vitamins from the greens. The remaining 25 percent of your plate can be quinoa with veggies or

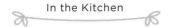

a raw veggie soup (try my Carrot Avocado Sun Soup, page 282). Hydration is key, so keep filtered water and coconut water on hand.

Glimmer Detox Sample Day

> *Upon Rising:* Warm water with the juice of half a lemon
> *Breakfast:* Green juice, then Quinoa Porridge (page 263)
> *Snack:* Goji Sunset Smoothie (page 257)
> *Lunch:* Rockin' Kale Salad (page 269)
> *Dinner:* Tomato & Garlic Salad (page 271)

Level III: The Glow

Turn up the glow volume! This plan is the most advanced of the prenatal detox options, yet it is still gentle on the body. It incorporates green juices, smoothies, raw salads, and sprouted nuts, legumes, and seeds. The Glow program offers an extra snack slot, which is allotted for an extra juice.

- *What's In:* Green juice, sprouted lentils, mung beans, quinoa, almonds, sunflower seeds, raw veggies, leafy greens, fruits (low glycemic), and smoothies.

- *What's Out:* Everything that's excluded from Glitz and Glimmer plus any cooked food. I would encourage everyone to try eating this way for the final week of your cleanse.

- *What You Can Expect:* Weight loss, glowing complexion, an increase in energy, and balanced mood.

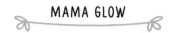

Continue your cleanse journal. Record what you consume, and how you feel. What changes have you noticed? How is your morale? What have you learned about your eating habits? What self-care practices have you incorporated during this process?

Breakfast: Drink a glass of room-temperature filtered water with the juice of half a lemon and liquid chlorophyll. Follow up with a 16-ounce green juice.

Snack: Try a 10- to 16-ounce smoothie here: Cherry Banana Split Smoothie (page 176) or Cacao Breeze Smoothie (page 259), or a handful of almonds.

Lunch: This could be a hearty raw soup, like Raw Hearty Chunky Chili (page 283) or Gazpacho (page 285).

Snack: 16-ounce green juice or coconut water.

Dinner: A light sprout salad with avocado and raw sunflower seeds, dressed with lemon and oil.

Glow Detox Sample Day

Upon Rising: Warm water, liquid chlorophyll, and the juice of half a lemon
Breakfast: Green Juice (page 262) or Mama Blood Builder (page 35)
Snack: Cacao Breeze Smoothie (page 259)
Lunch: Gazpacho (page 285), Green Juice (page 262)
Snack: Green Juice (page 262) or coconut water
Dinner: Avocado, Watercress, & Cumin Salad (page 268)

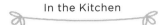

The Mama Blood Builder (2 servings)

This is one of my favorite drinks for prenatal health. I drank this every day when I was pregnant with my son. It gave me the antioxidant action and glyconutrient boost I needed to breeze through my day.

2 green apples
$\frac{1}{2}$ bunch kale
1 cucumber
3 celery stalks
1 cup parsley
$\frac{1}{2}$ to 1 whole lemon, peeled
1-inch piece of ginger
1 large beet (optional)

Process through a juicer and drink right away.

You're on your way to glowing from the inside out. Taking the time to slow down and cleanse your body of toxins, shed any excess weight, and fortify yourself with powerful nutrients will set the stage for fertile ground. Your body has everything it needs to make a healthy baby. In the next chapter, On the Mat, we'll explore making spiritual clearance with Mama Glow prepregnancy yoga. Part of the Mama Glow transformation includes mindfulness, meditation, affirmations, and movement. Roll out your yoga mat, grab your journal, and light a candle—this is going to be good!

CHAPTER 3

ON THE MAT

Making Clearance

Now that you're clearing your mind and life and detoxing your body, the time has come to explore the Mama Glow prepregnancy yoga and affirmations practice. In my practice I use specific yoga sequences and affirmations with clients to help them harness their inner dialogue and change the negative song in their head to something more empowering. It's a way to embark on pregnancy consciously. I call this chapter "Making Clearance" because the practices in it will clean the slate, so to speak, making us more open and receptive. Being receptive is what pregnancy is all about. "On the Mat" refers to a magical place where we step into our personal growth through yoga and movement: our yoga mat.

At this particular point in our pregnancy journey, we will be using yoga postures for detoxification and balance—especially twists and heat-building postures, both of which support cleansing. We also take a look at the divine feminine force, also known as Shakti.

Through meditation and affirmation practice, we will look at the power of our thoughts and how they affect our lives. An affirmation is a positive thought vibration that we can consciously create to shift negative thoughts. We'll develop a positive thought vocabulary because when we think it, we can achieve it. This emotional shift will set the tone for your journey toward pregnancy.

Practicing Clearance

I love to encourage women to be selfish, especially when trying/planning to get pregnant. By *selfish* I mean really taking time for yourself. Prepregnancy is a time when you need to make clearance for what you are about to receive. One of the Hindu Goddesses who can inspire us is Durga. Durga represents the warrior aspect of the Divine Mother, or Shakti. She is a powerful feminine force depicted riding on a tiger. She has eight arms, each carrying a weapon of consciousness. Her weapons that I love the most are her sword and her bow and arrow. The sword is about cutting through obstacles, and the bow and arrow are about targeting what you want. Since she is associated with clearance, Durga rules the bleeding phase of your monthly cycle.

Think about what in your life you are ready to cut out—what obstacles you are ready to clear. Also take a moment to think about what you are making room for—why are you clearing out at all? Then try some inspired movement, which will get your blood going and ground you in the present. Inspired movement is essentially dance, and it allows energy to move through your body. Often the movement I will suggest will mirror the affirmation or meditation.

The inspired movement for the clearance meditation is especially fun. I attended a conference with yogini extraordinaire Shiva Rea, and she had us use swords in an inspired movement practice. It felt really good to release pent-up energy and have the permission to just let go of some of our negative feelings like self-doubt and fear. We are going to do a similar exercise. You can do this whenever you feel like you need to let go of something in order to make space.

Clearance Movement Meditation

Start by standing with your feet hip-width apart. Bring your hands to your heart center and take a deep breath in through your nose, then sigh it all out through your mouth. Close your eyes, continuing to breathe in this manner. Do this a few times until you feel really grounded. Then imagine yourself in a field of tall grasses that are moving in the wind. Take one arm out in front of you and, pretending your arm is a sword, slowly start cutting the blades of grass. Do this for two minutes, then increase the intensity. Add your other arm to the practice. Start moving your body as your arms continue the cutting motion. Align your breath with the movement by inhaling deeply and, as you exhale through your mouth, say the word *HA!* while continuing to swing your arms. Imagine that you are cutting

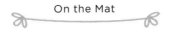

through some obstacles in your life, see them before you and cut right through them. This powerful movement meditation also gets the blood flowing and the heart pumping.

Allow yourself to release anything you are still holding onto that you don't need. Take long deep breaths, then wave your arm like a sword and cut through it. Cut through anything that is hindering you from getting pregnant. Name what you are ready to release. Say to yourself:

I am cutting through _____.

Do this practice for a minimum of ten minutes. If you'd like, you can create a whole ritual around it by lighting candles or burning sage. Turn on your favorite music if you like. When you are finished, take a seat on the floor, a pillow, or a chair. Close your eyes and visualize a clear field before you—a field of dreams and infinite possibility. What will grow there?

Planting Seeds of Renewal

Now that you've begun the process of clearance, it's time for renewal. You've opened yourself up and let go, so there is space to plant seeds for what you want to invite into your life. It's like unloading all your stuff at a massive garage sale. You see the potential for your home in a totally new light because now there is space for an interior makeover. Here's where we call in another face of the divine feminine—Lakshmi, the goddess of wealth, prosperity, generosity, creativity, and fertility. She is associated with uplifting mankind. This aspect of Shakti governs the ovulation phase of your cycle, the time of the month where you want to be still and receive. You can do this meditation following the Durga clearance meditation or you can perform them separately. I often find it feels best when I do both. First, I clear the space; then, I call in what I want. What do you want to manifest—or, as I like to call it, *womb-ifest?*

Womb-ifestation Meditation

Start in a seated position. You may be on the floor or in a comfortable chair with both feet on the floor. Sit up nice and tall. Start to breathe deeply, inhaling and exhaling through the nose. Do this for a few rounds until you start to feel grounded. Then place your hands on your knees and start rolling your hips in a clockwise circular motion.

Envision a seed, full of potential, ready to burst through the soil and blossom. It needs the right conditions—water, nutrients, and sunlight. Look at your own life and its seed potential. What have you suspended from coming into being because the conditions have not been right? What do you need in order to allow nature to take its course?

Start to rub your belly with both hands, acknowledging that this is the divine space that will house your baby.

Then envision yourself inside a lotus blossom suspended in a beautiful body of water. You are totally protected and provided for. Inhale and take your arms overhead; exhale and let them fall back to your sides. Then, placing one hand on your belly and one hand on your heart, say to yourself:

> *I am a being of expansive possibility.*
> *I live in a state of knowing, harnessing my intuition and wisdom.*
> *My soul dances in the uncertain and gives rise to perpetual creativity.*
> *My inner goddess co-creates with the universe.*

When you are ready to close out the meditation, draw your palms together in a prayer position, or mudra, at your heart. Keep your pinky fingers and thumbs pressed together while allowing your index, middle, and ring fingers to separate. With the base of the palms still touching, your hands look like a lotus blossom. The lotus blossom is symbolic of the womb. Holding your palms together in the lotus mudra, close your eyes and allow yourself to feel the creative energy within you. Visualize yourself holding all that you want in your palms.

The womb is the seat of creation, holding space for all that you want to call into your life, all that you want to womb-ifest. Harnessing the goddess energy helps us to get out of the head space and sink deeply into the womb space.

Repeat the womb-ifestation affirmations anytime you want to ignite your inner glow. You can say the four lines of affirmations all together as one affirmation or choose a line that resonates with you. Or feel free to write your own. For whichever you choose, write your affirmation down in a notebook or scrawl it on your bathroom mirror so you are reminded regularly that you are infinitely blessed.

Making Clearance Yoga Plan

Yoga helps women slow down and connect to what's happening in their bodies. It is a wonderful addition to an existing workout regime. Much like jogging, it's

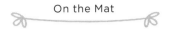

important to find the right pace for your yoga practice. It's about pushing yourself, but not about pushing to the point of injury, so pay attention to how your body responds to the movements.

The prepregnancy yoga plan should be implemented alongside your detox plan to maximize your glow power. When you follow the prescriptive guidelines for diet and get your body moving with yoga you will feel fantastic!

Postures like twists wring out our organs. These important poses aid the body in detoxification. Yoga twists stimulate digestion and facilitate the elimination of impurities and waste products from the body. Circulation of blood and of lymph is also promoted. The abdominal organs are squeezed during twists, stimulating the kidneys and liver, and forcing out blood filled with metabolic by-products and toxins. When the twists are released, fresh, clean blood enters these organs—bathing the cells in nutrients and oxygen. This is why the Making Clearance yoga practice that follows will include many twists.

Making Clearance Yoga Practice

Mountain Pose: This pose helps improve posture and strengthen thighs and arches of feet. It can also help relieve back pain.

How to do it: Start at the top of your yoga mat with your feet hip-width apart and your arms alongside your body. On the inhale, reach your arms up and overhead. As you exhale, bow forward over your legs and drop your head. If your hamstrings, calves, or lower back are tight this will feel especially good.

Standing Flamingo Kicks: This posture helps reduce water weight; tones thighs, glutes, abs, and arms; and releases the low back and shoulders. It also inverts and oxygenates the body for detoxification.

How to do it: Reach down to the floor and plant palms or fingertips on the mat at shoulder distance. Maintain your core strength by lifting the navel and low ribs toward the spine as you exhale and bring the right knee into the chest. Inhale deeply. As you exhale, kick your right foot into the air directly behind you, relax your jaw and strongly sigh, or vocalize as you wish to release old energy and bring in the new. Inhale to stretch longer toward a standing split, and exhale knee back into the chest. Do this 5 to 10 times, then switch sides.

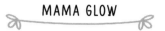

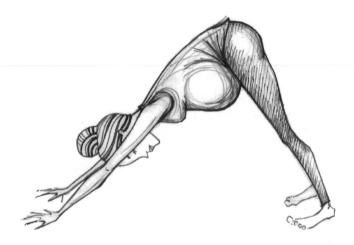

Downward-Dog Split: This pose strengthens arms; improves hip flexibility; tones the outer hips; stretches the hamstrings, calves, and thighs; and stimulates the liver and kidneys.

How to do it: From the Flamingo Kicks, plant your hands and walk back into Downward-Facing Dog Pose in which your body is positioned like an upside-down letter V (see image above). Spread palms and press hands and fingertips firmly into the mat; drop your heels toward the floor. As you shift your weight into the left leg, lift the right leg up and back behind you, flexing the foot. Point middle fingers forward to align the wrists. Square the hips and face, toes toward the floor, and lift your navel in toward your spine. Lift your leg higher toward a split, hold for five breaths, then switch sides.

Cat Back/Core Plank: This pose releases the lumbar spine, releases tension in the neck and cervical spine, tones the abs and thighs, and strengthens the arms.

How to do it: From Downward-Dog Split, exhale and sweep your right knee into the chest. Bring your shoulders over the wrists, and round up through the spine and hips. Relax the neck and drop the head toward the chest. Lift your navel into the spine, hold, and breathe for 3 to 5 breaths. Alternate with Downward-Dog Splits for the best heat-building results.

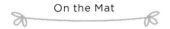

Twisted Lunge: This posture strengthens and stretches the knees, waist, ankles, groin, chest, and shoulders; stimulates the abdominal organs for detoxification; and increases spinal mobility, stamina, and lung capacity.

How to do it: During the last Cat Back/Core Plank, exhale and lightly step your right foot to the right thumb using the strength you've built in the previous postures. Lift your back thigh up to make space, then curl the tailbone down. Reach your arms up into a high lunge. Bring the palms together at your chest. Keep the back leg active and pull the navel in to move the front hip points back. Place your left elbow on or just outside of the right knee. Maintain squared hips, and roll the top shoulder back, deepening the twist from the heart slightly on each exhale. Take 3 to 5 breaths here, then spiral your arms to the floor, plant your hands, and return to Downward-Facing Dog Pose.

Child's Pose: This gentle stretch calms the brain, helping to relieve stress and fatigue; relieves back and neck pain; and stretches hips, thighs, and ankles.

How to do it: From Downward-Facing Dog Pose, kneel down to your mat, touch your big toes together, press your hips to your heels, separate your knees to hips' width, lay your torso down onto your thighs, back rounded. Rest your forehead on the mat, with your arms alongside your body with your palms facing upward. Breathe deeply into the back body for 5 to 10 breaths or more.

After your Child's Pose, return to hands and knees, and repeat the sequence from the Downward-Dog Splits to the end, this time on the left side of your body. After your last Child's Pose you can sit forward for a few minutes for a brief meditation. Place your hands on your belly and close your eyes. You may do this practice in the morning followed by the clearance affirmation practice, then in the evening with the womb-ifestation affirmation practice.

The benefits of this practice include burning calories; reducing water weight; toning thighs, glutes, abdominals, and arms; and releasing the lower back and shoulders. This series oxygenates the body for optimal detoxifying and supports stress release. It builds lean muscle to increase metabolism, preparing your body to be a perfect breeding ground. Find more yoga exercises to support your pre-pregnancy plan on www.mamaglow.com.

All this movement allows the release of energy blocks and leaves more space for what you want to draw into your life. What will you co-create with the universe? In the next chapter we will begin a process of journaling—sharing dreams, goals, and intentions—as well as establishing a contemplative practice to grow your spiritual stamina.

CHAPTER 4

IN YOUR LIFE

Holding the Space

Writing and reflections are a large part of my work with clients. One woman wrote for a year while we worked together and noticed that as she made subtle changes in her lifestyle, everything she wanted started appearing. Listening to her journal reflections helped me assess her internal progress. I could measure her results physically—through weight loss, endurance, and dietary shifts, but her internal landscape was made most visible when she would write. Holding the Space is all about honoring what you want and co-creating the life you desire. It's about aligning your actions with that desire.

Along with clearing out your life, detoxing, and setting intentions, you will now begin a process of "soul scribing"—also known as journaling—which will continue throughout the course of your pregnancy. You'll record your dreams, goals and intentions, and your answers to some of the self-reflective exercises in the book. In other words, you'll manifest your pregnancy.

It takes work to make change, to create the life you desire. How will you do it? These seven questions will help you map out your pregnancy vision and set your plan into action. Take a little time to soul scribe, answering the following questions either in your book or journal:

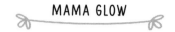
- What is my motivation for getting pregnant?

- How am I mentally preparing?

- What is my key emotional wound that needs healing?

- What plans am I putting in place?

- How have I tapped into my spiritual fortitude?

- What family and friends can I count on for support?

- What choices are in alignment with the life I want to lead?

Now let's take a look at the practices you can incorporate to develop your spiritual stamina, ease your mind, prepare your body, and access your inner diva. These will help you dial down the mental chatter and turn up the soul voice.

Create a Sacred Space: I'm a firm believer in setting up a space in your home to practice your meditation, yoga, and prayer. You don't need a whole room, just a small corner you can dedicate to yourself—a corner you will come back to on a regular basis to strengthen you spiritual muscles.

In my home, I reserve a place right in front of my bed for this purpose. It greets me when I wake up, and I am summoned to start my ritual. And throughout the day, I come back here to pray, plop my butt on a cushion, and sit in meditation.

One thing you can do to make your space feel more sacred is to set up an altar. I have altars all over my bedroom because I like to see something holy wherever I turn. Some cool altar elements include stones, crystals, symbols that resonate with you, seashells or other objects from nature, pictures of what inspires you, pictures of influential leaders who embody peace, fresh flowers, candles, or prayer beads. Whatever you choose should have meaning to you.

Establish a Seed Goal: The seed is a powerful metaphor for new life potential. A seed goal is similar to an intention but rooted in the deepest part of yourself. Your seed goal is a teeny tiny vision for something that, when in full bloom, will have a large impact in your life. If you are reading this book, my guess is that your seed goal is to get pregnant and have the best experience of your life. For instance, I have clients focus their attention toward conception—that precise moment. When we direct our energy, fruit is born.

Have Lots of ORGASMS!: That's right, I said it . . . and I mean it! You know that old adage, "an apple a day"? Well, it applies here, too. I don't really care how you go about it, as long as you feel safe, empowered, loved, respected, and SEXY!

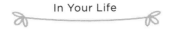

Acknowledge your primal appetite for sensual touch and the erotic. When women climax, the release of endorphins is very relaxing—it's like a tranquilizer. Orgasms regulate your appetite and reduce cravings for junk food. Those of us who want cookies and ice cream all too often may be craving a different type of sweetness . . . the kind that comes in the bedroom. Orgasms can also help with pain and stress management. So if you can't remember the last time you had one, you better get crackin'. If that doesn't get you glowing I don't know what will!

Love Your Body: When you get in the right relationship with your body—accepting your shape, quirks, and scars; celebrating your contours; and not trying to fit into anyone's mold—you will thrive! We women carry a legacy of loathing our body parts, and it's something we learn early in our lives. Our bodies deserve love from us. Through a healing and loving relationship with our bodies, we uncover an inner light and become more confident—and this shows on the outside. The body experiences so many changes during pregnancy. Getting to a place where you love and appreciate your body is key to really living the Mama Glow lifestyle. Show your body some love! Write a love poem for your most loathed body part. Gently massage areas of your body that could use more attention. Watch as these small changes begin to transform your relationship with your beautiful body.

Surround Yourself with Beauty: What you see is a reflection of what you are. When you can see beauty in all that is around you, it's a sign of inner beauty shining through. Place lovely flowers in pretty vases all over your home, open the curtains and let the light shine in, paint the walls a color that resonates with you. You want to feel good, beautiful, and elegant; that's part of the overall glow power. You deserve it, gorgeous!

Female Orgasm and Fertility

The uterus is marathon training for labor during arousal. It actually moves up and forward, in sync with the round ligaments that are attached to your vulva. This rocking movement, along with the shuddering pulsations of your orgasm, suck in semen as if through a straw. They help make a smooth and rapid trip up into the uterus, where one lucky sperm will meet your egg. The more we train these muscles and practice, the easier it will be for labor and birth. It's pretty simple: When you work out, your muscles get firm and strong. The uterus is no different. Do you really need more of a reason to stay in for a steamy Saturday night?

Take Out the Trash: Literally and figuratively! Clear any clutter or unnecessary disorder that shows up in your life. Resolving and dissolving emotional baggage can help you keep a clean heart. Clear out old clothes, clear your phone of some contacts you no longer need in your life—you see where I am going with this. I dump the trash monthly when I have my menses. It's a time when I am pensive and reflective, and I take stock of what is in my life that I can let go of. I clean the house like a madwoman. I empty out e-mail boxes and sort and shred snail mail. I also have a lot less tolerance for crap during this phase of my cycle.

Plop Down on a Pillow, Meditate, and Be Merry: Now that you've set up a sacred space in your home where you can sit in silence and tune inward, you can practice meditation and mindfulness. Deep breathing enables us to activate the parasympathetic nervous system and we have a release of endorphins in the bloodstream— happy hormones! This helps us to have peace of mind.

I told you this was going to be quite the journey, didn't I? Little did you know there would be so much to clean up beforehand. It's all about getting on track with what works for you so there is space to create the life of your dreams. Practice non-judgment and embrace every step toward your goal of optimal wellness. This is an educational process! So just keep glowing with the flow.

Glow Tips to Tune In

Elena Brower, mother, yogini, writer, love activist, healer, and founder of Vira Yoga in NYC, is one of my Mama Glow Icons because she really embodies what it means to go inside, clean up your crap, dispose of it, and beam bright. Elena has two essential glow tips for your pregnancy:

- **Learn to Love.** In every moment, love where you are, love what you're doing, and love the person who's next to you. That way there is no frustration in your body to distort your cells or the cells of your growing baby.

- **Cultivate Gratitude.** Every single day, thank someone for something. True gratitude is a true healer.

This concludes the first leg of your journey! You're now ready for pregnancy. You've done a lot of prep work. Now it's time to let that divine inner light guide you and your baby, trust your body, and let your glow shine through. Next stop: the first trimester.

part II

YOUR ABUNDANT PREGNANCY

FIRST TRIMESTER (WEEKS 1–13)

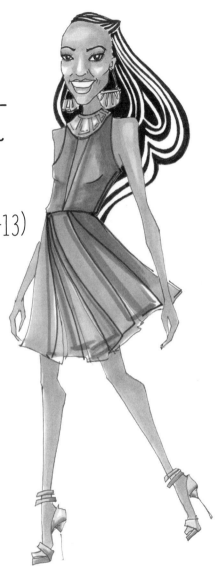

THE BUILDING BLOCKS

Baby Steps

Congratulations, girlfriend! Now you're pregnant. I remember when I first learned that I was having a baby. I was excited, confused, happy, and nervous all at the same time. I wondered if I was ready, if I was capable enough, smart enough, and resourceful enough to have my own child. I knew that eating right was half the battle, and I had that under control. But I had to learn how to be one with my body and my baby. I had to unlearn multitasking, and allow my body to slow down so I could actually feel what was going on deep within.

The first trimester is all about you, babe—your changing anatomy, your fluctuating emotions, getting enough rest (exhaustion is most common during this period), making sure you have spiritual guides in place, and taking care of your whole self. The second-trimester focus is on the baby. Your belly is finally showing, you have stronger nutritional demands, your baby is active and you can feel her communicating with you through movement. Best of all, you get your energy back! The third-trimester focus is on the birth: You are nearing the end of a transformational experience and soon you will be meeting your baby, so your mind focuses on the birth and nesting. Your body is more than prepared, so now thoughts and feelings surface about the big day.

In this chapter we are diving in to learn the principle of *listening to your body*. The first important skill is to learn to listen to what your body wants: adequate rest, food, and exercise—and lots of water. The more in balance you are from the standpoint of diet, fitness, and emotional well-being, the more you will be able to decode the messages your body is sending you. And the more you'll be able to stay on track with the healthiest pregnancy possible. Which brings us to baby fat, a topic we'll cover in this chapter. Gaining weight is an essential part of pregnancy, but you don't have to put on a ton to support the growing baby. So we'll talk about how to use glow foods to support a *gradual* and *healthy* weight gain. In Chapter 6, I'll hook you up with info on essential fats, vitamins, and minerals that will contribute to healthy fetal development. In Chapter 7, we will dive into the prenatal yoga principles that illuminate the Mama Glow. And in Chapter 8, we will explore sacred anatomy and shifting the way we perceive our bodies.

A Glance at Baby's Development in the First Trimester

- *Week 5:* Baby is at work forming major organs, including the kidneys, liver, and stomach—as well as the circulatory, digestive, and nervous systems.

- *Week 6:* Blood starts circulating and baby starts to develop eyes, ears, nose, cheeks, and chin.

- *Week 7:* Joints are starting to form and baby is developing arms and legs; 100 new brain cells are growing per minute!

- *Week 8:* The baby can begin to move arms and legs.

- *Week 9:* The embryo is now a fetus!

- *Week 10:* Arm joints are functional, bone and cartilage are forming, and vital organs are starting to function.

- *Week 13:* The intestines move from the umbilical cord to the fetus's tummy; baby is developing vocal cords.

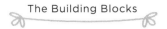

Mama's Development in the First Trimester

Just as a lot is going on with your baby in these first three months, a lot is going on with you as well! The number-one cardiovascular change in the pregnant mother's body is increased blood volume. This causes vasodilation of blood vessels, meaning the widening of blood vessels, resulting from relaxation of smooth muscle cells within the vessel walls. The stroke volume—the volume of blood pumped from one ventricle of the heart with each beat—increases. Pregnant women have up to 40 percent more blood in their bodies, which contributes to an increased heart rate. With this increase of water in the body, you'll see lots more mucus. You may experience more phlegm, or a runny nose from time to time—it doesn't mean you have a cold. Your joints may also become more mobile because of the increased volume of water in the body.

Overheating is an issue in the first trimester. Elevated levels of progesterone, combined with an increased metabolism, will raise your body temp a little during the entire pregnancy. Your hormones will be all over the place, and as a result of the fluctuation, you may feel uncomfortable at times. What I've come to realize, however, is that when we resolve our emotional matters, eruptions at the surface level are less frequent. I embraced my pregnancy emotionally and spiritually from the moment of conception. I felt a calling that was beyond my own personal desires to stay a single city girl. I recall the sacred pact I made with my baby. I was in the shower and I spoke out loud:

> Little being of light, I don't know who you are and what you will be in this world, but what I know is that you chose me. I don't feel ready but I promise you that I will ready myself for your greatness. I will cherish my body and protect you as you grow inside me, and I will do my best to raise you once you arrive.

What sacred pact are you making with *your* baby?

Top Three First-Trimester Challenges

Morning Sickness

Nausea can be a challenging symptom for many women during the first trimester. While I certainly experienced my own challenges during pregnancy, morning sickness was thankfully not one of them. I attribute this to the fact that I ate a

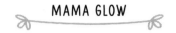
high-alkaline diet of glow foods with adequate protein at night. But not every mama will experience it this way.

Morning sickness appears to be caused by a combination of increased estrogen and progesterone levels, a heightened sense of smell, and excess stomach acids. Some women never get it; some go three months with morning sickness every day. Here are some ways to mitigate the morning sickness monster.

- Practice deep breathing, meditation, and yoga. Try to take a 30-minute walk in the fresh air every day.

- Consider possible emotional causes, including stress, uncertainty, and lack of support. Seek professional help if need be. Discuss your feelings with someone you trust.

- Try to remember to get up slowly out of bed and take your time in the morning.

- An infusion of grated ginger root may bring relief if you drink it while you're feeling nauseous.

- Tea made from fresh peppermint leaves can ease the stomach acids.

- Add more iron-rich foods—dried fruit, dark leafy green vegetables, and blackstrap molasses—to your diet.

- Grate lemon rind and sniff the fresh lemon to quell the queasiness.

- Eat a protein-rich meal or snack before bed to tide you over until breakfast.

- If you have no appetite, take 10 to 20 mg of vitamin B6 as a daily supplement.

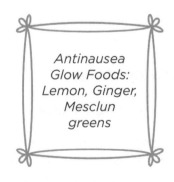

Antinausea Glow Foods: Lemon, Ginger, Mesclun greens

Lavender-Ginger Goddess Tonic
(4 servings)

This play on Caribbean ginger beer is an amazing tonic for getting through morning sickness. I recommend this to all my clients who have challenges with morning sickness. Lavender has been used to treat all sorts of stomach and digestive disorders. It soothes the lining of the digestive tract and promotes the secretion of bile, which helps the body digest fats. In addition, lavender can relieve gas pressure and constipation. Ginger is known to improve digestion, and alleviate gastrointestinal distress, migraines, and nausea. Plus it's anti-inflammatory.

1 cup peeled, finely chopped ginger
$\frac{1}{2}$ cup lavender flowers
$\frac{3}{4}$ cup raw agave nectar or honey
$\frac{1}{2}$ liter club soda
1 tablespoon lime juice
1 lime

Bring 3 cups of water to a boil in a saucepan. Add ginger and lavender. Reduce heat to medium-low and let ginger mixture sit in the simmering water for 5 minutes. Remove from heat and let sit for 20 minutes. Strain liquid through a fine mesh strainer. Discard ginger pieces and flowers. In a separate saucepan, boil 1 cup of water. Mix agave nectar or honey into water. Set aside to cool.

To make an individual glass, combine $\frac{1}{2}$ cup of lavender-ginger water with $\frac{1}{3}$ cup of sweetened water and $\frac{1}{2}$ cup of club soda. Add a few drops of fresh lime juice and a lime wedge to each glass. Store in the refrigerator in a bottle with a tight seal and sip when feeling nauseous.

Increased Urination

In the first trimester, you might find yourself heading to the bathroom more often than usual, especially at night. Shortly after you become pregnant, hormonal changes cause blood to flow more quickly through your kidneys, filling your bladder more often. Additionally, your enlarging uterus starts putting pressure on your bladder, causing you to leak urine when sneezing, coughing, or laughing. (Don't be alarmed; it happens to the best of us!)

As discussed earlier, over the course of your pregnancy the amount of blood in your body rises until you have almost 50 percent more than before you got pregnant. This leads to a lot of extra fluid getting processed through your kidneys—and ending up in your bladder. To help prevent urinary tract infections, take a bathroom trip whenever you feel the urge. If you're losing sleep due to midnight bathroom runs, drink less in the evening—especially fluids containing caffeine, which can make you urinate more. Don't skimp on the water intake, though; you and your baby need it. If you're worried about leaking, panty liners can offer a sense of security.

Panty liners will also catch any increased vaginal discharge, which is a normal part of pregnancy as well. The process that your body goes through when you become pregnant is called *implantation*. It's when the egg passes down through your uterus and attaches itself to the uterine wall. As a result of implantation, several changes takes place in your cervical area. Your cervix creates a mucus plug, which acts as a barrier between your baby and any outside bacteria or toxic substances. The increased flow of blood in your pelvic area causes old vaginal tissue and some harmless vaginal bacteria to pass through the vagina—exiting in the form of discharge. Normally the discharge during early pregnancy is an odorless, white, milky fluid.

> **Glow Tip:** Lean forward when you pee, to help completely empty your bladder.

One way to work with increased urination is to practice pelvic floor exercises, or Kegels. The term *pelvic floor* refers to the group of muscles that form a hammock across the opening of a woman's pelvis. These muscles, together with their surrounding tissues, keep all the pelvic organs in place so that the organs

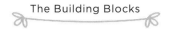
can function correctly. Practicing tightening and releasing of the PC (or pelvic muscles), which include the vaginal muscles, will give you more control when you laugh or sneeze.

Fatigue

Fatigue ranks pretty high among first-trimester symptoms. During early pregnancy, levels of the hormone progesterone soar. Progesterone is a female hormone for the regulation of ovulation and menstruation. Progesterone is produced by the corpus luteum of the ovary from the implantation of the embryo through the first eight weeks of pregnancy. For the balance of the pregnancy, the placenta takes over the production of progesterone. Progesterone then increases throughout pregnancy, and is necessary for the safe maintenance of pregnancy. But all this work makes the body tired. In a nutshell, more progesterone means more sleep is needed. At the same time, lower blood sugar levels, lower blood pressure, and increased blood production cause more work for your heart and other organs. The combination of all of this saps your energy. In this first three months, even night owls have a tough time staying up late enough to watch primetime television.

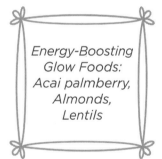

Energy-Boosting Glow Foods: Acai palmberry, Almonds, Lentils

So how do you combat fatigue? Quite simply—you don't. Go to sleep. Your body is working overtime, and you should give it the rest it's asking for. Make sure you're getting enough iron and protein (you will learn more about both in the next chapter). Try to make adjustments to your schedule to accommodate your need for more rest.

Pickles and Ice Cream

Most mamas experience their fair share of cravings. While the clichéd desire for pickles and ice cream may be extreme, you will likely find yourself wanting unusual foods in strange combinations. Relax—there is a biological reason for your cravings. Cravings are the result of a combination of physiological and emotional factors. When you experience a strong desire for a particular food, it's likely an indication that you are lacking the nutrients that this food offers. For instance, if you are craving sweet potatoes, your body may be lacking potassium. Cravings are actually your friend, honey. They aren't the problem, but rather the solution. They restore balance in the body. They're a blessing, a primal signal to get us back on track—especially during pregnancy, when we're concerned not only with our own nutrient balance but with our baby's, too! My approach is to appreciate the wisdom of the body—to listen to what the body is telling us through our cravings, and learn to pinpoint the underlying need rather than judge ourselves for having them. When we live with this attitude we learn a great deal about our bodies and what is working—and not working—in our diets.

I remember sending my boyfriend all the way across town to pick up tofu and seaweed sandwiches with sauerkraut from Angelica's Kitchen, an organic health-food restaurant in the East Village. It was the only thing I wanted to eat for weeks on end, it seemed. I examined my craving and realized that my desire for seaweed was my body signaling me that it wanted sea minerals like iodine. What I learned—and much of this crosses over to when you aren't pregnant, as well—is that when your relationship with food and with your body is in a healthy place, you don't get hung up on cravings.

Remember, pregnancy is not a competition. You don't have to worry about "being good" every day. Just focus on eating well *today*. Then, make that same commitment again tomorrow. Do this each day, and one day you will look back and say, "Wow, I have shifted my life." At a certain point, that choice you make each day becomes the *only* choice. Give yourself a break and enjoy a treat every now and again, but keep it balanced. Don't go overboard and have the entire pint of ice cream in one sitting. Choose healthier options that may satiate you. One of the reasons I love raw food is that you can almost always find a raw, vegan confection that approximates the sugary food you are craving, but it won't be loaded with butter, sugar, milk, and flour. My favorite is a chia seed pudding that I make at home. I discovered it at a local raw-food destination called Organic Avenue in NYC and have been in love ever since. It's a delicious way to get your essential fatty acids (EFAs). Chia seeds—a glow food—are a great source of dietary fiber and are rich in calcium, magnesium, iron, and antioxidants. They offer a complete protein to boot—what's not to love?

Vanilla Chia Pudding (8 servings)

Give my favorite a try! This pudding is a great omega-rich snack, and it makes for a healthy toddler food. It's still one of my son's favorite treats! You can adjust the sweetness by adding more or fewer dates to the liquid and blending prior to adding the chia seeds, starting with a minimum of five dates.

1 vanilla bean
7 cups nut milk (Brazil nut, hempseed, or cashew)
2 tablespoons vanilla extract
2 tablespoons cinnamon
5 to 7 dates
Pinch of sea salt
1 cup chia seeds

Split vanilla bean lengthwise and remove seeds. Set aside seeds and discard vanilla bean. Pulse all ingredients *except* the chia seeds in a high-speed blender. Place chia seeds in a large bowl, pour blended mixture over the chia seeds, and whisk to mix. Over the next hour and a half, continue to whisk the pudding periodically to be sure the chia seeds do not clump. You want a smooth, pudding-like consistency. Store in the refrigerator for up to four days.

Deconstructing Your Cravings

Learning to understand and deal with your cravings is a very important process. During my own pregnancy, I figured out how to do this for myself, and I use this same process time and time again with my clients. The steps will help you

How to Stop Eating When Full

For most of us, learning to eat when hungry is the easy part. But just like hunger, we can learn to tune in to our signals of *fullness*—and even begin to respect those signals. In order to respect your fullness, you have to be hungry to start with. If you aren't hungry, you are not going to be able to tell when you are full. Food tastes best if you are hungry and have worked up an appetite for it. You also need to be eating mindfully, focusing just on the process of eating. Being this hyper-focused won't always be necessary, but in the beginning you may need to pay a bit of extra attention to tune into the physical process of fullness.

determine what your body really wants, so you don't always fall prey to that desire for pickles and ice cream. The idea is to see if you are indeed hungry of if you are eating because you're bored, filling a void, or wanting to numb your emotions. This is a powerful process that will serve you well during pregnancy and beyond.

- *Step One:* When you feel a desire to eat, observe the emotions that come up with it. Do not judge, simply notice the emotions and use this as helpful data.

- *Step Two:* Drink water first! It's easy to mistake thirst for hunger. When you feel a craving coming on strong, drink a glass of water and wait about ten minutes to see if the craving subsides. If the craving is still there, or has come on even stronger, then you know your body does want food.

- *Step Three:* Eat a healthier version of the food you crave. A diet of refined foods and animal products can produce cravings for more of the same. To find your way back to balance, make a gradual transition from your current diet to one dominated by glow foods.

- *Step Four:* Cut back on the sweets, sugar! When we are consuming lots of sweets, it makes us crave more sweets as well as the polar opposite, salt. Want to have more sweetness in your life? Try meeting your craving with a little TLC. Take a nice warm bath with candles and lavender essential oil, get your nails done, or go for a massage to meet that emotional need for sweetness.

- *Step Five:* Spot-check for foods and/or lifestyle factors that may be the real source

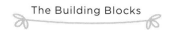

of cravings. In other words, see if you are stressed—relationally, at work, or financially. If so, you may find yourself reaching for bon-bons, cakes, or other rich desserts. If you are craving hard candies, popcorn, or other crunchy carbs this may signal some pent-up energy that needs an outlet. Try exercise such as vigorous yoga or brisk walks.

- *Step Six:* Ask yourself, "If I eat this, will I be satisfied?" If the answer is "yes," then have a small portion of the food. If the answer is "no," try one of the practices listed above instead.

- *Step Seven:* Learn and respect your limits. Honor the sensation of fullness.

With all this talk of craving, I bet you want to know what each of your cravings actually means. Well, below I share the craving decoder. This is based upon the five flavors, which define organ relationships with specific foods and how flavor affects an organ. This is based in traditional Chinese medicine and is a useful tool to understand where you may have imbalances and what the cravings are saying about your internal state.

The Craving Decoder		
Flavor	**Organs**	**Internal State**
Sweet	Spleen, stomach, and pancreas	Calming/soothing, filling emotional void: cravings indicate blood sugar imbalance, need for emotional balance, excessive protein consumption
Salty	Kidneys and bladder	Softening: cravings indicate a need for minerals, coping with stress
Bitter	Heart and small intestine	Drying effect: cravings indicate a need to cut through fat, or middle organ sluggishness
Spicy/Pungent	Lungs and large intestine	Dispersing: cravings indicate mucus buildup in the lungs and large intestine. Pungent foods help to induce perspiration and disperse mucus. Spicy cravings may indicate zinc deficiency and that you need help regulating your body temperature.
Sour	Liver and gallbladder	Astringent and emptying: cravings indicate chemical imbalance requiring a neutralization of acids in the body

The Skinny on Fasting

The most relevant message about nutrition for pregnant women can be summarized in two words: Eat well! During pregnancy, more than at any other time in a woman's life, it is vitally important to eat lots of healthy food and to avoid skipping meals. Your body is undergoing many changes to allow for the growth of your fetus and to prepare you for labor, delivery, and lactation. Many of these changes increase your nutritional requirements. These requirements don't change when you skip a meal. Fasting creates more hunger and more cravings. When you finally give in to these extra-strong hunger pangs, you may end up bingeing on less desirable foods than you would have chosen had you eaten when you first felt the urge. Avoiding meals causes the body to behave as if it's facing a famine; your metabolism begins to slow down. Rather than burning calories to lose weight, your body actually conserves calories and retains weight.

The moral of this story is: Don't fast during pregnancy! Instead, try snacking on plant-based foods between meals to keep your insulin levels low. Insulin is a hormone that is needed to convert blood sugar, or glucose, into useable energy. You want to keep your blood sugar consistent and want to avoid major spikes and falls in glucose levels. Plant-based, whole-food snacking is also preferable because it means fewer chemicals, less sodium, and less fat. Look for nourishing, on-the-go recipes in the recipe appendix at the end of the book.

The first trimester is an exciting time marked by subtle changes. It's crucial to set your new patterns in place now. Baby steps toward your optimal glow requires a commitment to making proper food choices. In Chapter 6, In the Kitchen, we will dive into your prenatal pantry and get you all stocked up from staple foods to equipment.

CHAPTER 6

IN THE KITCHEN
Your Prenatal Pantry

How do we develop an authentic relationship with our food? As expectant and new mothers, how can we make sure our diet is in step with nature, while meeting the needs of our busy modern lives? I had a nonfunctional kitchen when I was pregnant, which meant that I was forced to purchase fresh food every other day. I wouldn't wish those circumstances on any mommy-to-be! However, I made it work. Whatever your circumstances, you can, too. I was already a bit of a health nut, but I went deeper because I really wanted to understand what my body required and eat super-well for my baby.

So what *should* we be eating to maintain optimal spiritual and emotional well-being—and for our budding bundles of joy? Forming a healthy relationship with food is about accepting nourishment in many forms—receiving it not only from the foods we eat but also from all the good things that come our way in our lives. Our experiences in life have a way of feeding and nourishing us that can't be counted in calories. After I have a great hang session with one of my girlfriends I always feel full. And spending time with my beloved makes me feel so satisfied that food is nowhere on my mind. The quality of our experiences can be so nurturing that they keep us from falling into addictive patterns around food.

The dietary advice I dish out is focused on a plant-based diet that's grounded in vegan and raw cuisine. Raw foods are vegetables, fruits, nuts, seeds, and some grains that have not been cooked. They are kept at temperatures below 108 degrees, which preserves their naturally occurring enzymes. These enzymes aid in the digestion and assimilation of nutrients in our food. While some experts say enzymes are preserved if food is kept below 115 degrees, I play it safe and keep it under 110 if I'm preparing raw food. I found that incorporating raw foods into my prenatal diet sustained my energy levels and satisfied me. And my nails and hair grew like weeds!

I'll let you in on a little secret: it wasn't part of some grand plan to become a raw foodie during my pregnancy. It was sort of an accident (I say "sort of" because I've come to believe there's no such thing as accidents). While I was pregnant, my boyfriend and I lived in what we New Yorkers call a studio apartment and what anyone else in the U.S. would consider a closet. Ours was not a full kitchen, which for me was a huge deal because I love to cook. I've done it since I was a kid, and I'm damn good at it, too! I love shopping for ingredients and prepping meals, so the nearly nonexistent kitchen was a challenge, but it didn't set me back one bit.

I lived two blocks from the first Whole Foods to pop up in New York City, so trips there became a part of my daily routine, along with weekly visits to the Green Market in Union Square for my microgreens, sprouts, and seasonal fruits. I also indulged in lavish lunches at three of my favorite raw-food spots. Each day I would prepare fresh food for myself and pack snacks for my "mobile pantry." And as I already mentioned, I would also regularly send my boyfriend out to get me Asian seaweed and tofu sandwiches. I've been vegetarian since age 12 and knew that a healthy vegetarian/vegan pregnancy was totally feasible if I was eating the proper glow foods. I am not saying that everyone should be vegan or go raw, but most people need to include more plant foods in their diet.

My suggestions are intended to help complement and enhance your current diet. If you incorporate the dietary practices—eat mindfully, embrace glow foods—and find a way to weave in the lifestyle tips that suit your needs and goals, you'll grow a healthy baby and you'll get the ever-sought-after Mama Glow!

You Are What You Eat

The most significant change you can make in your eating habits is to be mindful of the quality of foods you eat. Eating organic, locally grown, seasonal foodstuffs is best. Local foods taste better and have lower environmental impact because they traveled less distance from farm to market than the conventionally grown produce that is shipped from all over the world. We already went over this: Do your best to avoid dairy products altogether, and steer clear of those with bovine

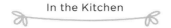
growth hormones. Generally avoid pesticides, hormones, and antibiotics in your food. They pass through the mother's bloodstream at an alarming concentration relative to the baby's size.

But what's a diva mom to do when there are so many choices and so little time? It's tempting to buy into the convenience of eating packaged foods like potato chips, pastries, and frozen meals. The unfortunate reality is that packaged foods have hidden ingredients, many of which we can't even pronounce. Most are full of sodium, sugar, and all the wrong types of fats—yuck!

When you eat processed foods your body leaches vitamins and minerals from your tissues in an effort to transition out of an acidic state and into a more alkaline state. Vitamin and mineral depletion equals malnourishment, which leads to lackluster skin, chipping nails, and moodiness—among other things. None of which is part of the glow plan! Chemical processing should not be in your vocabulary, ladies! Your food should be fresh! Lots of fresh fruits and vegetables will build strong blood and healthy cells. What you eat breaks down into what your body uses to grow your baby. You can't build a mansion out of sand. You need strong, solid bricks to build with. Wouldn't you rather give your body—and your baby—the best building blocks available?

Go Green!

I first became fascinated with tender greens as I began to study medicinal herbs as a youngster. My interest ultimately grew into the study of plant physiology. The vibrational energy of organically grown plants is beneficial beyond measure. I wasn't always so gung-ho about greens. I remember my mother would make sautéed Chinese broccoli for dinner and I refused to eat it, so much so that I remember sitting at the dinner table alone, pushing the greens around the plate with my fork, long after my mom and sister had finished eating. I would never have guessed that I would have a deep love affair with greens when I grew older. Plain and simple, greens make you glow. If I don't eat them every day, I feel "a little off." Eat at least 1 to 2 fresh salads daily made from dark leafy greens or bitter greens like arugula, mizuna, mâche, mixed baby greens, watercress, and dandelion. Cover them with all of your favorite glow-food toppings: avocado, carrots, almonds, cranberries, hempseeds, and bean sprouts. Our ancient ancestors used to eat about six pounds of greens daily! Just so you have the visual, six pounds is like a *grocery bag* full of greens. Can you imagine eating an entire grocery bag full of greens? I guess one could assume they were constantly foraging, or just plain bored. But whatever the case, they were eating a lot more greens than we are today. In fact, according to a study conducted by Cornell University, most people need to *triple* their weekly servings of dark green leafy vegetables to meet the one-serving-per-day recommendation. Remember: When you're green inside, you're clean inside. The more leafy greens you eat, the more efficient your elimination. Greens are even more powerful, because they are charged with ions that bond with toxins in our tissues to carry out waste.

Greens are rich in minerals—including iron, calcium, potassium, and magnesium. They're also a great source of vitamins, including K, C, E, and many of the B vitamins. They provide a variety of phytonutrients including beta-carotene, lutein, and zeaxanthin, which protect our cells from damage and our eyes from age-related problems, among many other benefits. Dark green leaves even contain small amounts of omega-3 fats. They help to regulate blood sugar, break down fats, and cleanse the blood. This is key! To help break down the fat from a heavy meal, add a side of greens.

Dark leafy greens that are great for cooking include collards, kale, mustards, chard, and spinach. One of the major benefits of eating cooked greens is their relationship to vitamin K. Vitamin K regulates blood clotting, helps protect bones from osteoporosis, reduces calcium in arterial plaques, and helps prevent diabetes. A cup of nearly any cooked green provides at least *nine times* the minimum recommended intake of vitamin K. Several cups of dark salad greens provide the minimum all on their own.

> **Glow Tip:** *Vitamin K is a fat-soluble vitamin, which means it dissolves in fat , and is absorbed by the small intestine. Unlike water-soluble vitamins, vitamin K doesn't need to be replaced each day. Make sure to put oil-based dressing on your salad, or cook your greens with olive oil.*

I ate so many greens during my pregnancy that I was nearly photosynthesizing. I glimmered with sheen from the chlorophyll coursing through my system. People wondered what the secret was to my healthy pregnancy skin and tresses . . . well the cat is out of the bag, my friend. Chlorophyll is an antioxidant, antimicrobial, and anti-inflammatory, and it's alkaline so it naturally balances out any acidity in the body and contributes to a brighter, smoother complexion.

Sassy Sautéed Collard Green Ribbons (4 servings)

One of my favorite ways to eat greens is lightly sautéed. This is a Southern-inspired collard green preparation that takes just minutes to make, looks vibrant, and tastes great. The key to this recipe is the *light* sauté of the greens. These greens are at their best when sautéed just five minutes. They retain more nutrients that way, not to mention the vibrant green color. Most people overcook their greens, or "cook them to death" as my grandmother would say!

It speeds the cooking process to use a chiffonade technique, slicing the greens into long, thin strips, creating ribbons (see below for instruction). This technique can be used on all types of robust greens, including kale, mustard greens, chard, and more. Note that if you can't find good-quality fresh leafy greens, look for organic frozen greens. Equal in nutrient density, they are tasty and better than not having greens at all.

2 bunches collard greens
1 tablespoon olive oil
2 garlic cloves, crushed (optional)
Sea salt, to taste
$\frac{1}{4}$ teaspoon crushed red pepper

Wash the greens thoroughly and chop off the end of the stems. Take 3 collard leaves at a time, stack them together, and roll them up width-wise. Hold in place against the cutting board and make $\frac{1}{4}$-inch slices through the collard roll and place ribbons in a large bowl; continue cutting the remainder of the greens in this way. When you are done you should have a heap of collard ribbons.

Heat olive oil in a large pan on medium-high heat; swirl the pan to cover the entire surface with oil. Add the crushed garlic if using and cook for 2 minutes before adding the collard greens. Sprinkle about 2 tablespoons of water over the greens, stir, and then cover to cook for 4 to 5 minutes. Remove the lid, sprinkle with sea salt and red pepper, and toss the greens again. Serve immediately.

Keep It Colorful!

Get creative! Keeping a rainbow of colors and variety of textures on your plate is a great way to ensure full-spectrum nutrition. This is a great time in your pregnancy to use a variety of cooking techniques and preparations. Don't be afraid to show off! Go for the widest variety of fruits and veggies and do your best to avoid white foods: white sugar, white flour, white rice, and white potatoes. These foods are low in nutrients and contribute to high blood pressure, obesity, diabetes, mood swings, and fatigue because they spike your blood sugar levels, wreaking havoc on your pancreas. The last thing you want right now is to be sleepy and in a bad mood! Color also makes meals more visually interesting. When you take the time to make a beautiful plate of food, you are honoring yourself and your energetic requirements. You are crafting a healthy relationship with food for you and your baby when you eat in balance.

Drink Up!

It sounds simple enough, yet it's difficult for many of us to drink as much water as our body requires. We learned back in grammar school that our bodies are composed of about 70 percent water. Since we are composed mostly of water, we need to quickly replace it when it's depleted. The body needs water to perform its metabolic processes.

We may carry our cute little water bottles around town, but how much are we actually *drinking* from them? Dehydration is far more common than we realize. Most of us have no idea when we are dehydrated. Warning signs include a strong sense of hunger, headache, dry mouth, dry skin, thirst, dark-colored and odorous urine, fatigue, and weakness. If you don't stay hydrated, your body won't function well. Boosting your water also helps increase your metabolism. If you're worried about excess water weight, remember you're likely to retain more water (causing swelling in ankles, feet, hands, and face) when you're not drinking enough because your body perceives that there is not enough water so it starts to retain it.

I cannot tell you how many mamas I've had to coax into drinking water over the course of my time as a pregnancy consultant. Maternal dehydration can lead to prematurity, as well as a reduction in amniotic fluid volume associated with fetal growth restriction. There can be major complications for mama associated with dehydration including increased heart rate, increased respiration (which means decreased intake of oxygen), decreased perspiration, decreased urination,

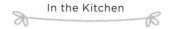

increased body temperature, lethargy, headaches, nausea, and muscle cramps. During pregnancy, when the volume of liquid in your body increases, your water intake is crucial. Your baby is encased in a bag of amniotic fluid that is affected by your levels of hydration. Uterine contractions and premature labor are associated with poor hydration. You want the baby to stay in the womb for a minimum of 36 weeks, but 40 to 41 weeks is ideal.

To keep your water intake in check, remember the 8 by 8 rule: drink eight 8-ounce glasses of water daily (for a total of 64 ounces). You need at least 2.5 quarts of fresh water daily, roughly a half gallon, and even more if you are eating processed foods because they require a lot of water to digest. Coffee, black teas, soft drinks, and power drinks are excluded from your requirements because they promote dehydration and can elevate blood pressure, which is very serious in pregnancy. It can restrict the baby's growth, cause premature contractions, and cause complications for the mother later. Alcohol should be avoided, although small amounts of alcoholic beverages like wine are sometimes used therapeutically during labor (that's another chapter, though!).

So what should you drink your water from? Believe it or not, bottled water is not as safe as we once thought. Harmful chemicals in plastic can leach into the water, especially if the plastic is exposed to heat. Avoid drinking water from plastic bottles that have been sitting in the sun. My favorite solution is carrying a stainless steel water bottle, and the brand I love is Klean Kanteen.

If you are not a fan of plain water, mix it up by adding lemon, orange, or cucumber slices to give it a little flavor. This a much better option than choosing commercially available flavored waters, many of which contain sugar and artificial flavorings. If you live in a place with old pipes or funky water, consider installing a water filtration system. It cuts down on the expense and chemical danger of bottled water. Choose herbal teas like raspberry leaf tea, which contains an alkaloid that promotes uterine muscle tone, and nettle tea, which fortifies the blood with iron (see recipes in the appendix). Or check out my favorite tea supplier, Tavalon, for some cool herbal blends. You can drink your herbal tea hot, or brew it ahead of time and keep it chilled in your water bottle—mama's choice. Whatever you do, keep on sipping!

Calcium, Magnesium, and Zinc . . . Oh My!

Let's talk numbers! Every day you need at least *80 grams of protein,* which is about 2.82 ounces of your preferred source. You also need at least *6 servings of*

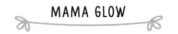
complex carbohydrates, and a total of *2,500 calories.* Thirty percent of your daily calories should come from fat.

A daily intake of complex carbohydrates in the form of vegetables and whole grains or fruit is needed for a problem-free pregnancy. Glucose, the basic stuff of carbohydrates, is the main source of energy drawn on by the fetus. Fats that contain essential fatty acids, such as flaxseed oil, hempseed oil, and avocado, are critical for the development and functioning of the baby's nervous system. While whole foods are the best source for all of the essential nutrients, in some cases supplements can be a great addition to a healthy diet.

Get Crazy for Calcium

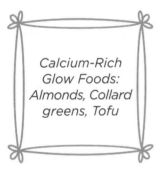

Calcium-Rich Glow Foods: Almonds, Collard greens, Tofu

A substantial transfer of calcium occurs between the mother and the fetus throughout pregnancy, allowing for the baby's bones and teeth to form. In the first six months, you store up calcium in your own bones. When your baby's skeletal growth reaches its peak in the last three months, the fetus draws on your store. So you better stock up, girlfriend! This is when the consumption of high calcium–containing foods such as dark leafy green vegetables must be increased, since calcium deficiency will damage the mother's teeth and make her bones brittle. I've heard crazy stories of our great-great-grandmothers back in the day losing teeth during pregnancy—well, this is why!

Calcium cannot be absorbed without magnesium, they are BFFs. Take them together. Best to take them at night because the combination will make your mind and muscles relax. You are loading up on minerals, which means your body will have what it needs on hand for overnight tissue repair.

Iron Woman

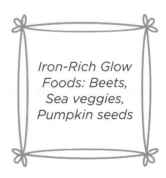

Iron-Rich Glow Foods: Beets, Sea veggies, Pumpkin seeds

The demand for iron, which is essential for blood formation, also increases during pregnancy because the maternal blood volume increases and the fetal red blood

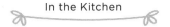

cells have to be developed. In addition to red meat, iron is available in whole-grain products and vegetables. However, iron of plant origin is not as well assimilated as iron of animal origin. So be sure to ingest raw foods high in vitamin C, including lemon, lime, kiwi, kale, red bell peppers, or fresh thyme, which helps your body absorb iron, during the same meal. Supplements of 30 mg of iron daily during the second and third trimesters is recommended.

Fantastic Folic Acid

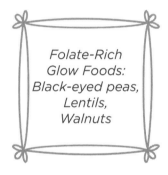

*Folate-Rich
Glow Foods:
Black-eyed peas,
Lentils,
Walnuts*

Folic acid, also known as vitamin B9, promotes the development of the fetal central nervous system and prevents developmental defects of the neural tube (including spina bifida). Folic acid can be found in vegetables including okra, broccoli, Brussels sprouts, asparagus, leafy greens; legumes including black beans, black-eyed peas, lentils, pinto beans, and edamame; and fruits like orange and papaya. We do not always get enough folic acid to meet the requirements of pregnancy. Additional intake is necessary in the months before pregnancy and during the first trimester. As I mentioned in the prepregnancy chapters, taking a prenatal vitamin including folic acid is critical when you are thinking about having a baby. This is because folate is required by your baby very early on in pregnancy, before many of us even realize we are pregnant. The recommended dose is a minimum of 400 mcg daily. Plant-based diets tend to be high in folic acid, but to be safe, always take a supplement. You will want to take folic acid throughout the pregnancy and have your blood work checked out at a prenatal visit to be sure your levels are on point.

Mad for Magnesium

When you're pregnant, magnesium helps build and repair your body's tissues. A severe deficiency during pregnancy may lead to preeclampsia, characterized by high blood pressure and protein in the urine after 20 weeks of pregnancy. It can lead to poor fetal growth, and even infant mortality. Due to the high blood pressure factor, mothers with preeclampsia are confined to bed rest during their last trimester.

The great news is that magnesium and calcium work in combination: magnesium relaxes muscles, while calcium stimulates muscles to contract. Research suggests that proper levels of magnesium during pregnancy can help keep the uterus from contracting prematurely.

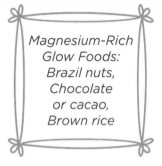

Magnesium-Rich Glow Foods: Brazil nuts, Chocolate or cacao, Brown rice

Magnesium also helps build strong bones and teeth, regulates insulin and blood sugar levels, and helps certain enzymatic function. Research indicates it may help control cholesterol and irregular heartbeats. Magnesium is also helpful in reducing leg cramps. Many of my prenatal yoga students have taken calcium/magnesium supplements for leg cramping and general relaxation, with great success. You need about 350 mg of magnesium daily. In case you didn't know, this mineral is found in a food very dear to many of us: chocolate! So really, ladies, there is no excuse to be deficient.

From A to Zinc

A woman's requirement for zinc increases during pregnancy, mainly because the mineral is needed during development of the embryo and fetus. Zinc is required for the production, repair, and functioning of DNA—the baby's genetic blueprint and the basic building block for cells. This essential mineral also helps support your immune system, maintains your senses of taste and smell, and heals wounds.

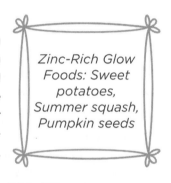

Zinc-Rich Glow Foods: Sweet potatoes, Summer squash, Pumpkin seeds

Zinc is necessary for the functioning of more than 300 different enzymes, which means it plays a role in a great number of bodily activities. Some of those activities are critical during pregnancy, because they involve embryo and fetal development as well as infant growth. Zinc supplementation helps with the accumulation of lean tissue mass, which is beneficial to a child's health. The daily requirement for zinc is 15 mg.

Alpha and Omega-3s

Omega-3s are a type of polyunsaturated fatty acids. They are found in various foods, including nuts, seeds, plants, and in the fatty layers of cold-water fish like salmon, mackerel, herring, and sardines. Polyunsaturated fatty acids are one of four types of fats that your body gets through your food. Though omega-3s are called *fatty acids,* they are actually very good for you and are a necessary component for both mental and physical health. Omega-3 fatty acids are often referred to as *essential fatty acids*, because they cannot be produced by your own body but must instead be obtained through foods.

DHA is a type of fat that is mainly found in fatty fish. It is crucial for the development of the brain, nervous system, and retinas. Some DHA can be made from another fat called alpha linolenic acid, or ALA, which can be found in flaxseed, flaxseed oil, walnuts, and soybeans. Choosing these foods regularly, and avoiding foods containing the trans fats that can interfere with DHA production, can help to enhance DHA production. Another option is to use a vegan-friendly DHA supplement produced from microalgae.

You may be wondering when to begin taking omega-3 supplements or to increase your natural intake of the fatty acid through food. As I said earlier, omega-3 is actually something that you should be including in your diet on a regular basis before pregnancy. During pregnancy, it is recommended that you get at least 250 mg of omega-3s every day. However, omega-3 oils are especially important during the final trimester of pregnancy. It is during this time that your baby uses omega-3s to form approximately 70 percent of her brain system. So omegas are literally brain food.

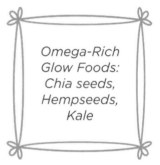

Omega-Rich Glow Foods: Chia seeds, Hempseeds, Kale

When eating a healthy and balanced diet it's possible that you would consume your daily supply of omega-3s within the scope of a day. Flaxseed oil, hempseed oil, or algae oil can be taken in lieu of fish oil. This supplementation is a necessary addition to the diet as 85 percent of women are deficient in omega-3 DHA and EPA, another critical omega-3 fatty acid. I suggest Udo's Oil or Flora brands.

Glow Tip: *Our brains shrink between 3 to 5 percent during late pregnancy. There's good news, though: the brain is restored to its normal size within a few weeks or months postpartum. If this doesn't drive home my point about eating your brain food, I don't know what will. Make sure to take your omega-3s to help replace the stores your baby is using.*

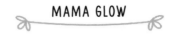
Big on B12

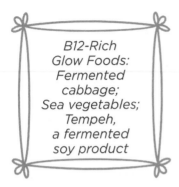

B12-Rich Glow Foods: Fermented cabbage; Sea vegetables; Tempeh, a fermented soy product

Vitamin B12 is crucial early in pregnancy, when a deficiency can cause brain or central nervous system abnormalities in your baby. As it is difficult to get adequate B12 from vegetable sources absorbable through the gut, vegans can best obtain B12 from sublingual tablets placed under the tongue or at the gum line, which absorb directly into the bloodstream.

Protect with Protein!

The USDA's average requirement of protein for women ages 31 to 50 is 46 g per day. An additional intake of 10 g ($\frac{1}{3}$ ounce) of protein a day during the entire pregnancy is recommended to build up, maintain, and regenerate body tissue in both the fetus and mother.

Insufficient protein can lead to low blood sugar levels by mid-morning and fierce sugar cravings, so it's important to get the protein you need. We know 16 ounces equals one pound, so 2 ounces is a fairly small amount of protein—much less than what we are taught we need to eat in order to maintain a healthy balance. Simply adding a cup and a half of cooked lentils to your daily routine will tack on the extra protein. In the last trimester, needs for protein, iron, and calcium increase to accommodate the baby's rapid growth. In the final six weeks, the baby gains about half a pound per week, so monitor your intake of these nutrients. Extra protein is necessary for brain maturation and musculature, extra

Protein-Packed Glow Foods: Quinoa, Hemp seeds, Spinach

calcium for well-developed bones. Because breast milk is low in iron, the baby stores iron in its system to sustain itself until solids are introduced between six to ten months. If the baby doesn't have sufficient iron stores, it may need supplements or solid food before it's developmentally ready. We will talk about this more in Part III.

Inca Protein Queen Salad (6 servings)

Check out one of my favorite protein-rich salads here. This really helped to keep me satisfied during pregnancy. It contains many of the aforementioned nutrients so it's a wonderful addition to your diet and so easy to make.

For the dressing:

$^2/_3$ cup olive oil
2 tablespoons mustard
Juice of 1 lime
Sea salt and pepper, to taste

For the salad:

2 cups cooked quinoa
3 tablespoons whole flaxseeds
Pinch of sea salt
One 8-ounce packet of tempeh
3 tablespoons nama shoyu soy sauce
1 teaspoon olive oil
$^1/_2$ pound baby arugula, rinsed well
2 cups frozen corn, thawed
$^1/_2$ onion, diced
3 tablespoons hempseeds
$^1/_2$ cup chopped cilantro
1 avocado, peeled, pitted, cut into cubes

Whisk all dressing ingredients together in a small bowl and set aside.

While the quinoa is still warm, mix in the flaxseeds and a touch of sea salt; then set aside. Cut the tempeh into $^1/_2$-inch-thick strips and place on a plate. Pour soy sauce over the tempeh, marinate for at least 10 minutes. Heat a saucepan over medium-high heat and lightly coat it in olive oil. Place the tempeh in the pan and sear on all sides; it should be a nice caramel color after 7 to 10 minutes. Once cooked, cut the tempeh into cubes. In a large salad bowl place the arugula, corn, onion, hempseeds, cilantro, and quinoa, and lightly toss. Add the tempeh and avocado, and top with dressing. Mix thoroughly and serve. Enjoy!

Complex Carbs Run the Show!

Complex carbohydrates are composed of long chains of sugars bound within fiber. Complex carbohydrates are found in fruits, vegetables, nuts, seeds, and grains. Some examples of foods high in starchy complex carbohydrates include bread, cereal, whole-grain brown rice, pasta, potatoes, dry beans, carrots, and corn. Green vegetables like green beans, broccoli, and spinach contain less starch and more fiber. All grains include carbohydrates, but you want to indulge in the less starchy variety as they prevent a spike in blood sugar.

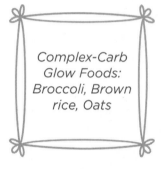

Complex-Carb Glow Foods: Broccoli, Brown rice, Oats

Complex carbohydrates should be a major part of your diet. About half of your daily calories should come from carbohydrates—mostly from vegetables, grains, cereals, and fruits. None of your daily calories should come from simple carbohydrates like table sugar. It's okay if you have a sweet tooth, but you want to be sure that when indulging in sweets you choose the best options—meaning sugar alternatives—and cut back on table sugar in general. There are a ton of healthier alternatives to sugar that you can explore.

Simple carbohydrates are made up of one or two sugar molecules linked together. Examples of simple carbohydrates include glucose, fructose (fruit sugar), sucrose (table sugar), and galactose (the sugar found in milk). Simple sugars are used as ingredients in candy, ice cream, cookies, and other sweets. Plus they occur naturally in fruits and, in lesser amounts, in vegetables.

Complex carbohydrates also contain sugars, but ones with longer, more complex chains. Because of this, the human body takes longer to break them down. These sugars have to be freed from fiber to be released into the bloodstream. The process of releasing sugars from foods starts when we begin chewing, aided by the enzyme amylase found in saliva. Once digestion has begun in the mouth, the process continues when the food reaches the small intestine where the sugar is slowly released. In other words, the process of sugar absorption takes a while for complex carbs like brown rice and vegetables, compared to simple sugars like bagels and other white breads that burn fast—and burn out. Slower absorption allows the body time to use the carbohydrates, and as a result fewer of the carbs turn to fat. You also don't have to worry about a sugar spike and crash when you eat more complex carbs rather than simple sugars.

Complex carbs mean you can get the fueling benefits of carbohydrates while gaining weight the *healthy* way, throughout your pregnancy. Another key advantage of complex carbohydrates is the fiber content. Fibrous foods have more bulk than low-fiber foods, warding off hunger and keeping you satisfied. A fiber-rich diet is also beneficial in alleviating and preventing constipation, an unpleasant side effect of pregnancy that plagues many women.

> ***Glow Tip:*** *Carbs are the feel-good foods,*
> *as they increase the amino acid tryptophan,*
> *which elevates the neurotransmitter serotonin.*
> *Serotonin boosts your ability to concentrate*
> *and, when tired, allows for more restful sleep.*

Ohhhh How Sweet It Is . . . Not

Move over sweet stuff, we are taking a detour to the not-so-saccharine side of sugar. Sugar is essentially fuel for cells—it stimulates metabolic activity—but it provides zero nutrition. What I mean is that the sugar in marshmallows, for example, offers energy for your cells—but you and I both know marshmallows are devoid of nutrition. Such simple sugars enter your bloodstream within minutes of being ingested, where they elevate blood sugar and insulin. This in turn can cause mood swings, excess weight gain, mineral depletion, heart disease, and arthritis, among other disorders. Unfortunately, the standard American diet is loaded with sugar. Even those of us who are doing our best are *still* ingesting a lot of it. That said, we can do a lot to control how much sugar we eat and in what forms. First and foremost, it's best to avoid white sugar, which is processed, refined, devoid of fiber, acidifying, and taxing to your pancreas. I would also recommend staying away from synthetic sweeteners, many of which contain aspartame. Aspartame is an aggressive neurotoxin that is associated with about 90 side effects, including headaches, brain tumors, memory lapses, and grand mal seizures—yikes! That's so not a part of the glow plan, sister!

Aspartame contains two isolated amino acids—spartic acid, which literally excites cells to death (they become overstimulated and die), and phenylalanine, which lowers the serotonin levels in the brain, causing feelings of depression. If you know you have a sweet tooth, don't be in denial of it. There are ways to embrace it more healthfully. Try integrating sweet-tasting foods into your diet, like sweet potatoes, pears, and cinnamon. These foods are soothing to the pancreas and can satisfy the body's craving for sweetness. For healthier alternatives to sugar try the following:

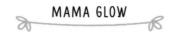

Agave Nectar: Although I no longer use this sweetener, I think it is important to mention. Agave comes from the same plant that gives us tequila—the blue agave. Native to southern Mexico, the plant produces agave nectar, which is 90 percent fructose and much sweeter than sugar. Its viscosity is somewhere between honey and maple syrup. New research is emerging about agave being similar in composition to high fructose corn syrup, which is a definite no-no, so I have chosen to eliminate it from my diet and introduce my clients to other options. You will find some recipes that call for it, but I also offer an alternative.

Brown Rice Syrup: Brown rice syrup contains 50 percent soluble complex carbohydrates, derived by culturing cooked rice with enzymes (usually from dried barley sprouts). It takes two to three hours to be digested, resulting in a steady supply of energy.

Coconut Nectar: Coconut nectar is low on the glycemic index, full of vitamins, minerals, and amino acids. It is made from the sap of the budding flower that will eventually form a coconut. It has a rich, nutty, butterscotchlike flavor.

Local Honey: Honey has more calories and carbs than refined sugar. Yet raw honey has medicinal benefits and contains enzymes and small amounts of minerals and B-complex vitamins. Local honey is a must as it inoculates your immune system with pollen from local plants, offering resistance to seasonal allergies. Since it is sweeter than sugar you can use less of it.

Maple Syrup: Grade B maple syrup, which is darker than the more popular grade A variety, also contains more vitamins and minerals than honey.

Stevia: Made from an extract of the stevia plant, stevia boasts zero calories, rates zero on the glycemic index, and is about 300 times sweeter than sugar—so only the tiniest amount is necessary. I happen to enjoy stevia as an alternative sweetener and have even convinced my mom to make the switch from the evil artificial sweetener she previously used for her iced tea. That said, some people are sensitive to stevia's aftertaste.

Yacon Syrup: Native to the Andean region of South America, yacon syrup is pressed from the roots of the yacon tuber and is glucose free, tastes like caramel, and is full of antioxidants and potassium. This alternative sweetner also promotes the growth of healthy bacteria in the colon.

Cumin-Cinnamon Roasted Sweet Potatoes (8 Servings)

My cumin sweet potatoes will soothe the pancreas and satisfy your desire for a sweet sensation. This dish is excellent alongside collard green ribbons and marinated tempeh.

2 1/2 pounds sweet potatoes (about 4 medium-sized)
1 tablespoon ground cumin
1 tablespoon ground cinnamon
1 1/2 teaspoons black pepper
1 teaspoon sea salt
2 to 3 tablespoons coconut oil

Preheat the oven to 375 degrees. Thoroughly wash the sweet potatoes and cut into 1/2-inch chunks, leaving the skin on. Spread the sweet potatoes across a cooking sheet or large roasting pan. Sprinkle the cumin, cinnamon, pepper, and sea salt over the potatoes; then pour the oil over them and mix until they are evenly coated. Sprinkle them with 2 tablespoons of water so they retain some moisture as they cook. Place in the oven. Turn the potatoes every 15 minutes or so. Roast for 40 minutes or until nicely browned.

Just a Touch of Fat

What do we need fat for? A lot of things: vitamin D production, cholesterol for maintaining the integrity of your cells, sex hormone production, good healthy skin, and to cushion organs.

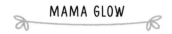

Fats are an important part of your diet, but not all fats are created equal. The goal is to make sure you are getting adequate good-quality fats and minimizing the intake of bad fats.

Some fats (and the fatty acids they contain) are particularly important during pregnancy because they support your baby's brain and eye development—both before and after birth. Fats also help the placenta and other tissues grow, and studies show that some fats may help prevent preterm birth and low birth weight.

Let's get acquainted with our fatty friends. There are four types of fatty acids found in food: monounsaturated, polyunsaturated, saturated, and hydrogenated. A fat is made up of a combination of fatty acids, so individual fats don't typically fall into just one of these categories. Palm oil, for example, contains about 50 percent monounsaturated and 50 percent saturated fat. Sound complicated? I'm about to make your life a whole lot simpler. Because for the most part, you can follow some simple guidelines when choosing your fats.

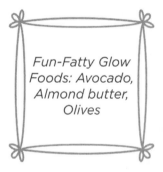

Fun-Fatty Glow Foods: Avocado, Almond butter, Olives

Monounsaturated fats are found in safflower, olive, canola, and peanut oils, as well as in olives, avocados, nuts, and nut butters. They're considered good fats because they're best at lowering cholesterol. These fats are no good when cooked, however. They are completely unstable when heated. When cooking, I advise all of my clients to give up the canola and peanut oils and use coconut oil for high heat and cold-pressed olive oil for lower temperatures. I also recommend never reusing oil that has already been cooked. To get your monounsaturated fats through foods, try almonds, peanuts, macadamia nuts, cashews, hazelnuts, and olives.

Polyunsaturated fats are beneficial, too. They contain the omega-3 fatty acids (like our friends DHA and ALA, both of which are crucial for the healthy development of your baby) and omega-6 fatty acids. Omega-3s are found in flaxseed oil and canola oil, while omega-6s are found in sunflower, cottonseed, corn, and soybean oils. Foods that deliver polyunsaturated fats include walnuts, Brazil nuts, sunflower seeds, sesame seeds, chia seeds, and hemp seeds. Many monounsaturated and polyunsaturated fats also contain vitamin E, an important antioxidant often missing in the typical American diet—something very important to skin elasticity and healthy nails and hair.

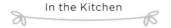
Saturated fats fall into the bad-fat camp. They're mostly to be avoided. Saturated fats are found in high-fat meats, whole milk, tropical oils (such as palm kernel and coconut), butter, and lard. A vegan diet will exclude most saturated fat, unless you are getting it from tropical oils. Tropical oils can be used in moderation. My favorite is coconut oil, which I love for skin care, cooking, and making some of the nice vegan desserts you will find in this book. This oil protects the body from free radicals and is antifungal as well.

Hydrogenated and partially hydrogenated fats (the polite way of saying trans fats) are to be avoided at all costs. These are fats that have been heated for a long time and at a high temperature. They are found in fried foods and some kinds of margarine. They're also used in some packaged foods, including crackers, cookies, and chips, to extend shelf life. The process of hydrogenation (turning a liquid vegetable oil into a solid fat) creates trans fatty acids (TFAs), which are toxic fats that enter cell membranes, block utilization of essential fatty acids, and impede cell functionality. TFAs also cause a rise in blood cholesterol. They interfere with your metabolic processes by taking the place of a natural substance that performs a critical function. Read the "Nutrition Facts" label on processed foods to find the amount of saturated and trans fat in a product. You should know a lot of packaged foods won't list that they contain TFAs. There are two reasons why foods containing hydrogenated oils may be labeled trans-fat free, or list 0 g trans fat on the label. First, items that list partially hydrogenated oils in the ingredients but contain less than 0.5 g of trans fat *per serving* are considered by the government to be trans-fat free. A good example of this would be commercial peanut butter, which contains a tiny amount of partially hydrogenated oil to prevent separation. The problem with this definition, though, is that if you eat more than the stated serving size, those fractions of a gram add up.

A diet high in saturated and trans fats can raise your cholesterol and may put you at risk for heart disease later in life. Studies show that saturated and hydrogenated fats may be linked to other health problems, too, such as cancer and diabetes. There's even some evidence linking trans fats to lower birth weights in newborns and a higher risk of having a small-for-gestational-age (SGA) baby.

Don't beat yourself up if you indulge in a bag of savory chips or a side of French fries on occasion. We all do it! I'm a sucker for good fries with truffle salt . . . well, anything with truffle salt! Just make it the exception rather than the rule, aiming for healthy fats as much as possible. I like to get my fat from avocado. Slicing it up and adding it to a salad can make any salad feel more substantial. I also make

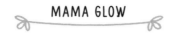

my own salad dressings, using part extra-virgin, cold-pressed olive oil and part flaxseed oil, which is a great way to get the best quality daily fat. Here are some guidelines to help you determine how much of these oils you should eat in a day:

- At least 2 teaspoons (10 ml) nutritious vegetable oil such as sunflower oil, thistle oil, extra-virgin olive oil, pumpkin seed oil, flaxseed oil, for example, for salad dressings.

- At most 2 teaspoons (10 ml) cooking oil, such as coconut or olive oil for cooking and hot meal preparation.

Goddess Herb Dressing (8 servings)

Try my simple herb salad dressing, loaded with EFAs, to give you some of that Mama Glow I keep talking about. This dressing works well tossed over greens, or steamed or sautéed veggies, and can keep well in the refrigerator. It should not be heated as it contains flax oil—which should never be heated, because it can easily oxidize.

6 tablespoons olive oil
2 tablespoons flaxseed or borage oil
2 tablespoons chopped fresh parsley
2 tablespoons fresh squeezed lemon
     juice
2 garlic cloves, peeled and chopped
1 teaspoon dried basil, crumbled
¼ teaspoon dried crushed red pepper
Pinch of dried oregano
Pinch of sea salt

Process all ingredients in a high-speed blender for a smooth dressing. If you like a chunkier dressing, chop the ingredients by hand and then whisk together in a bowl.

Get Your Glow On!

Bringing your focus to locally grown (when possible), seasonal, organic (when possible) whole foods will help to maintain an optimal hormonal balance, producing the Mama Glow you're looking for! The list in the sidebar offers a rundown of the glow foods I embraced during pregnancy and what I recommend moms indulge in before, during, and after pregnancy. As you move through the rest of the book, you will find more of my delicious recipes. If you give them a try, I can almost guarantee you will be obsessed with quite a few of them before you finish this book.

Good nutrition prompts your baby to grow normally and to store sufficient fat for stabilizing blood sugar levels, allowing him to sleep more easily and nurse more contently. Poor nutrition increases susceptibility to stress—and chronic stress takes its toll by rapidly depleting B and C vitamins along with trace minerals essential for normal fetal growth and a healthy maternal blood volume.

Get Equipped!

One of the biggest challenges for people changing their diet and lifestyle is proper preparation. If you are going to run a marathon, you probably want to train for it. You'll need proper running shoes, maybe a cute little outfit, a trainer or running partner, and some sweatbands just to look cool—all before you begin. You're not just going to roll out of bed and show up to the race expecting to do well! Similarly, when you decide to switch up some of your less-than-healthy habits for better ones, you need the right equipment—the right setup so you can succeed. If you don't have a well-stocked refrigerator and cabinets, you're going to feel like you don't have options. That, in turn, will drive you to make poor

My Go-to Glow Foods

- *Grains:* Quinoa, millet, brown rice, amaranth

- *Beans:* Chickpeas, black beans, kidney beans, mung beans, lentils

- *Nuts:* Almonds, Brazil nuts, walnuts, pecans

- *Seeds:* Pumpkin seeds, chia seeds, hempseeds

- *Vegetables:* Beets, shiitake mushrooms, sweet potatoes, garlic

- *Leafy Greens:* Kale, collards, mustards, chard, arugula

- *Sea Vegetables*: Arame, kombu, kelp, dulse

- *Fruits:* Grapefruit, blueberries, avocados, acai, goji berries

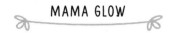
choices. If you invest in some good equipment, you can do wonders in the kitchen, making healthy food in minutes. Check out some of my must-haves when it comes to kitchen gear.

Food Dehydrator: A low-temperature "oven" used to gently dry fruit or prepare raw dishes, creating heartier textures while maintaining nutritional integrity. Excalibur is the brand I recommend. I have a five-tray model at home and it works wonders. If you have more space, I say splurge and get the nine-tray version.

Food Processor: This appliance is used to assist in the chopping and shredding of vegetables and in the grinding of nuts and seeds. A mini-prep or standard-size food processor will cut your prep time in half. I have a Cuisinart, but any brand will suffice.

High-Speed Blender: A blender is a device that pulverizes solids and mixes ingredients into a smooth texture. Any commercial-style blender with a 2-horsepower (or higher) motor will do just fine. The Vitamix is the Cadillac of blenders. Blendtec is also a fancy brand. While these are cool toys for the kitchen that will last for years, you don't need this type of blender to make the recipes I've listed. A $29 blender will also do the trick.

Juicer/Juice Extractor: A machine that separates the juice from the fiber of vegetables and fruits. The Hurom Slow Juicer and the Green Star brand are the most efficient on the market. The Breville fountain works pretty well, too. I lived on fresh grapefruit juice during my first trimester. If you don't have a juicer, no problem, a blender works in most cases. If you're not a pulpy kind of gal, you can strain out the pulp.

Miscellaneous Kitchen Tools

8- or 10-inch Chef's Knife: Any chef will tell you that the most important piece of equipment is a good knife. A sharp knife is essential. You are less likely to cut yourself with a sharp knife than a dull one. A great knife also means you can move more quickly and with more precision, reducing prep time.

Chinois: If you're not into the cloth thing (see nut milk bag/cheesecloth section on the next page), then you can use the chinois. A chinois looks like a giant funnel, made of fine mesh for straining.

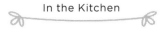

Green Cookware: Most brand-new cookware is relatively healthy. Damaged cooking surfaces can cause a few health problems, however. Recycle any aluminum, copper, or steel pans that have scratched-up cooking surfaces, as the metal can leach into your food and make you sick. Also, Teflon-coated pans are problematic. At high temperatures, Teflon will release a gas that has been shown to kill birds and give people flulike symptoms—yikes! Now that you're cooking (and eating) for more than one, it's a great time to upgrade and get green cookware. What I mean by *green* is cookware made without Teflon or aluminum. This kind of cookware is good for you to cook with—and good for the planet as well. There are many products on the market now, but I'm a fan of the old-school stuff: stainless-steel pots (which are fully recyclable once they wear out), cast-iron skillets (which offer a bit of iron via the cooking process), and glass cookware (which doubles as a storage container for refrigeration).

Mandolin Slicer: A mandolin is a cooking utensil that produces thin, precise slices of fruits and veggies. Make sure to get a model with a safety guard to protect your hands.

Nut Milk Bag/Cheesecloth: This is one of my favorite handy tools for straining nut milks. The nut milk bag is made of a very fine mesh that only allows liquid particles through. So if, for instance, you are making almond milk, you can strain the milk and save the pulp.

Vegetable Peeler: I don't believe in giving yourself extra work. A vegetable peeler makes things so much easier than peeling with a knife. Use the veggie peeler to skin produce like cucumbers, carrots, and the like.

Stock Up!

Now that you have the equipment you need, it's time to pack your cabinets and refrigerator with glow foods that will get you through your pregnancy. Pick and choose from the following list to create a kitchen full of staples. Happy shopping!

Acidic Flavorings

Citrus Fruits: Lemon, lime, grapefruit

- **What to Look for:** Organic, ripe (note that a ripe lime will look yellow)

Fermented Veggies: Sauerkraut, pickles, Korean-style kimchi

- **What to Look for:** Organic, unpasteurized

Vinegars: Apple cider, balsamic, rice vinegar

- **What to Look for:** Organic, raw, unpasteurized, unfiltered, packaged in glass

Healthy Fats

Fatty Fruits: Avocado, olives

- **What to Look for:** Organic, raw, ripe

- **Notes on Fatty Fruits:** When eaten with sweet fruits, fatty fruits will slow the release of sugar into the bloodstream. Avocados are best when they have little to no smell when you cut them open, as odor indicates they have gone rancid. Olives are best when they are ripe. Find varieties packaged in purified water or cold-pressed olive oil, either with or without sea salt added.

Nuts: Almonds, macadamia nuts, Brazil nuts, cashews, coconuts, pecans, hazelnuts, pine nuts, pistachios, walnuts

- **What to Look for:** Organic, raw, unsalted

- **Notes on Nuts:** If your macadamia and pine nuts are yellow-to-orange in color, that means they've become rancid—toss them. To preserve your nuts keep them in the refrigerator. My

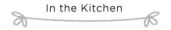

refrigerator is full of nuts on the condiment shelf. Also, nuts should be soaked and/or dehydrated for easier digestion.

Nut and Seed Butters: Almond butter, tahini (sesame seed butter), coconut butter, pumpkin seed butter, hempseed butter

- **What to Look for:** Organic, cold-processed (raw), unsalted, salted with sea salt

Oils: Coconut oil, flaxseed oil, cacao butter, hempseed oil, olive oil, sesame oil, avocado oil, pumpkin seed oil, borage oil

- **What to Look for:** Organic, cold- or stone-pressed, unrefined. Packaged in a dark glass bottle

- **Notes on Oils:** Flaxseed oil must be stored in the refrigerator immediately after purchasing or it will become rancid within hours. Olive oil is best when stone-pressed and made from ripe olives. Look for the term *cold-pressed* on the label. Untoasted sesame oil is best—look for this term on the package. Store any oil blends in the refrigerator.

Seeds: Chia seeds, flaxseeds, sesame seeds, hempseeds, pumpkin seeds, sunflower seeds

- **What to Look for:** Organic, raw, unsalted

- **Note on Seeds:** Seeds are easy to digest and don't require soaking.

Savory & Salty

Salt: Celtic sea salt, natural solar-dried sea salt, Himalayan salt, premier pink sea salt, flower of the ocean

- **What to Look for:** Sun-dried, unbleached, noniodized

Salty Ingredients: Nama shoyu (organic, unpasteurized soy sauce), unpasteurized miso, olives packed in sea salt, celery salt, whole-leaf dulse, dulse flakes, kelp flakes, nori

- **What to Look for:** Organic, wild harvested, unpasteurized, non-bleached

- **Notes on Salty Ingredients:** While not actual "salts," these ingredients will lend a salty taste to a dish. Raw nori is black, toasted nori is green.

Sweetness

Dried Fruit: Dates, apricots, figs, coconut, prunes, bananas, raisins, mulberries, tomatoes, goji berries

- **What to Look for:** Organic, unsulfured, sun-dried

Fresh Fruits: Apples, grapes, bananas, kiwi, tomatoes, pears, berries, mangos, sweet peppers, melons, pineapple, cherries, plums, squash

- **What to Look for:** Organic, ripe

Honey: Alfalfa, blueberry, clover, manuka, orange blossom, sage, tupelo, wildflower

- **Honey Categories:** Comb honey (honeycomb), liquid honey (extracted), creamed honey (granulated), chunk honey (comb honey in a jar with liquid honey poured over it)

- **What to Look for**: Organic, wild-crafted honey is best. Local is preferred and can be purchased at farmers' markets. Choose unfiltered and unheated.

Other Sweeteners: Coconut water, fresh stevia, agave nectar

- **What to Look for:** Organic

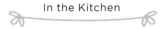

Mama Glow Checklist:

Take a moment to see what steps you need to take in order to make your pre-natal pantry the bomb.

- ☐ Load up on green, leafy veggies. Make sure to have salad and/or cooked greens twice daily.

- ☐ Keep it colorful. Eat lots of carrots, beets, greens, tomatoes, and blueberries. The more colorful your foods, the more full-spectrum vitamins, minerals, and antioxidants you're getting.

- ☐ Drink lots of water. Remember the 8 by 8 rule: at least 8 glasses of 8 ounces each.

- ☐ Get your prenatal vitamins (if you aren't already taking them).

- ☐ Eat multiple small meals throughout the day to keep blood sugar balanced and to prevent heartburn.

- ☐ Fortify your diet with adequate iron, protein, calcium, and potassium through glow foods.

- ☐ Get your plant-based proteins through quinoa and hempseeds.

- ☐ Chuck the sugary stuff and replace it with agave nectar, maple syrup, honey, or brown rice syrup.

- ☐ Bring on the fats! Coconut, flaxseed, and hempseed oil, plus olives and avocado.

- ☐ Get set with your equipment—remember your knives, pots, food processor, blender, and dehydrator.

- ☐ Stock it up! Fill your pantry and refrigerator with glow foods—dry ingredients, spices, fruits, and veggies. Try new things and find out what your favorite go-to glow foods might be.

You're all stocked up with fresh and dry ingredients, you've got all the equipment you need, and you have a better understanding of what to look for when you are purchasing ingredients and equipment. Get cozy at your local grocery or farmers' market because you will be spending a lot of time there while you've got this bun in the oven. The next chapter, On the Mat, explores the Mama Glow prenatal yoga principles, and the grounding and energizing postures and affirmations to help guide you to a place of total awareness.

CHAPTER 7

ON THE MAT

Prenatal Yoga Principles

When I was pregnant with my son, I remember searching for a place to practice yoga where I felt empowered. I was active and athletic so I could go to a regular class but I wanted to be with other pregnant moms as well. What I discovered was a lot of prenatal classes that should have been called "prenatal naptime class for expectant moms"—not prenatal yoga. I made a promise that I would teach prenatal yoga that made women feel strong, capable, and divine. That's what you will find here in *Mama Glow:* a yoga practice that honors the wisdom of your body and prepares you for pregnancy and birth.

The beauty of yoga is that you can practice it anytime and anywhere. Not to mention it offers a plethora of health benefits including improving circulation, firming of the skin, strengthening of the muscles and connective tissue, and stimulating lymphatic flow. Yoga promotes peace of mind, helping ground us in the present. It helps us connect with our higher self—our inner diva. Mama Glow prenatal yoga is a sequence of postures designed to develop strength and flexibility in the body as well as awareness and openness on a mental and spiritual level. It employs principles such as mindfulness, gratitude, turning inward, and opening. This section will focus on standing postures and affirmations to ground you in the experience of pregnancy. During this first trimester you may also feel more tired than you ever have in your life—so these postures will help to energize you as well.

The Seven Key Principles to Mama Glow Yoga

I'm big on living by principles and understanding what really ignites the glow from within. As I look back on my pregnancy journals and the work I have done with mommies-to-be, there are seven key principles that I feel really promote the lifestyle that I prescribe. I still follow these principles as a mother with a young boy and strongly believe in incorporating them into my life to flex my spiritual muscles.

So let's get familiar with the seven key principles.

Flexibility: This means living with balance and suppleness of mind, body, and attitude. It means being open to change. When you are pliant, you can easily go with the flow. This is so important during pregnancy, and even more so during labor. Being flexible is important because shit happens, my friend. You don't want to be so regimented that you can't flow with the unexpected changes that may arise. Flexibility teaches us the lesson of letting go. You're not always going to be able to control the circumstances, so why not learn how to relax, let go, and flow?

Gratitude: See each moment of your pregnancy and your baby's life as a total gift. This pregnancy experience will never happen again in the same way. Pregnancy is an exclusive party and you, my dear, are on the coveted guest list. I'm not saying you can't have off moments, I'm just saying that embracing an attitude of gratitude will help you focus on the blessings and miracles unfolding all around you—making you more content with your pregnancy and your life as a whole.

Intention: Be clear about what you want during your pregnancy and in your life. Whenever we set out to do something—whether it's to do the laundry or bake a cake—we have a goal in mind. Make a conscious practice of setting intentions for what you want to experience during this pregnancy and birth. Set a clear vision of what you want, and align your actions with the fulfillment of that intention. Intention is important because it helps us practice accountability in co-creating our reality. When we speak what we want, we communicate that with the universe. Your only job is to live a life that is aligned with the achievement of your goal; the rest will unfold on its own.

Glow Power: This is unconditional and expansive love, living fruitfully and healthily, celebrating your pregnancy, and sharing your abundant light with those around you—infecting others with your glow. Glow power is really about celebrating life and finding the magic in all your experiences.

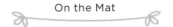
Mindfulness: This is really about stepping into the now, not being stuck in the past or worrying about the future. This means that you turn off your cell phone, log off Facebook, and take some time to connect with what is happening within you. Pregnancy is a finite period, and you only get to experience this pregnancy once, so savor each moment of it.

Opening: It's just like it sounds: opening up means allowing yourself to expand in heart, mind, spirit, and in the body. You become an ever-expanding portal for your baby's entrance into the world. Envision yourself giving birth to your baby. Your body was made to do this! Trust in yourself, woman.

Tuning Inside: Tuning inside means turning your senses inward. This is especially helpful for labor, when all of your energy needs to be focused on what is happening in your body. Visualization techniques are key! Being able to go inside yourself will allow you to hear the voice of your primal power guiding you through the birth.

These principles are woven throughout the On the Mat yoga practices in this book. The Mama Glow yoga practice includes some traditional yoga asanas, or poses, woven together with what I call "movement meditation"—movements inspired by dance and other traditions. They help us to drop deeply into our bodies and make the hips more pliant to facilitate an easier pregnancy and birth. I encourage you to explore movement meditation daily. Turn on your favorite music, dim the lights, close your eyes, and begin to let your body guide you to dance. This is about getting comfortable with your body and expressing yourself. I find this especially helpful to do for a few minutes before beginning my yoga practice. When I teach I always allow space for this before we begin the class. Some music suggestions include classical Indian music, African drumming, electronic, jazz, or house music.

Just Breathe!

Here in the first trimester, the time has come to bring focus to the breath. Breath is the bridge that overlaps the conscious and unconscious, because the respiratory system is both voluntary and involuntary. Your breath will follow every state you are in, whether it be anxiety (shallow breathing) or relaxation (slower, fuller diaphragmatic breathing). The amazing thing about the breath is that you can manipulate it voluntarily to encourage different states. If you are stressed out or afraid and your body is naturally breathing shallowly, you can use awareness to change the rhythm. You may take a big long inhale through the nose and a long exhale through the mouth, for example. This will facilitate a response in the body that signals the brain to stop producing stress hormones and instead to activate a relaxation response. Breathing through the nose and exhaling through the mouth tends to light up the primal pathway. I encourage exploration of this type of breathing with an open throat and relaxed jaw. Remember, your mouth and throat are one end of a channel that leads to the pelvic floor and birth canal—the sacred passageway. When the mouth and throat are relaxed, so are the pelvic floor and sacred passageway—something important to remember on the road to giving birth.

Meditation offers an opportunity to enter a quiet space within through single-pointed focus. This altered state we can achieve through breath work is actually a shifting of our brain waves from beta to alpha states. I think of this as switching from first into second gear. Later we will explore how this can be helpful during your labor.

But we're getting ahead of ourselves, mama! Here in the first trimester, we're just going to practice breathing. I know for some it may sound weird to "practice breathing," since we all know how to breathe already. But when I say *practice* I mean bringing *conscious attention* to your breath. I am going to share one great breathing exercise that I love. It's called *Ujjayi*, or Victorious Breath. I like to call it "Mother of the Sea" or "Mermaid" breathing, because it sounds like the rolling waves of the sea pulling back from the shoreline and crashing again along the sand. Benefits of practicing Mother of the Sea breathing include balancing the nervous system, expelling stale air from the lungs, and slowing rapid brain waves, which increases focus. If visualizing the beach takes you into a relaxed state, go for it. Either way, imagine the sweet sounds of the boundless sea flowing within you. Here are the steps to practice:

1. Find a comfortable seated position.

2. Inhale slowly and exhale fully once or twice. Draw the breath in through the nose and, with your lips gently closed, allow the breath to flow out through the nose.

3. After a couple full breaths, begin a slow inhalation, filling the belly and chest.

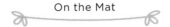
4. Keeping your mouth closed and relaxed, contract the throat slightly to create a soft hissing sound as you exhale through the nose, completely emptying the lungs.

5. Repeat steps 3 and 4. Make each inhale and exhale long and slow, until your breath sounds like the ocean tide. Repeat at least five times.

Get Your Om On!

Yoga asanas and inspired movement have a way of tuning people in to what is happening in their bodies. Yoga helps people wake up to life, becoming aware of their inner world and outer surroundings. It's my preferred method to teach body awareness because the tools translate right from the mat to the delivery room. Yoga is effective because it helps you to get out of your mind and into your body, bringing awareness that is critical in preconception, pregnancy, and labor. Remember, we are going for proper alignment, so do what works for you and your body right now. Don't worry if you can't do the full expression of the pose. In pregnancy yoga, we align poses starting with the hips. In any posture you will make sure your hips are in proper position first, and then you will align your legs, feet, shoulders, and neck from there. It doesn't need to be about perfection, it's about finding the sweet spot in your body and reaching a little beyond. It's about seeing where you can take your body today. Don't force yourself or "should" yourself here, just do what feels comfortable and right. Use the illustrations to follow along. I'm going to show you how to get those hips flexible, for a more comfortable pregnancy and labor.

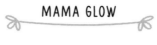

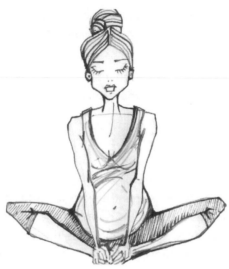

Shakti Seat (or Cobbler's Pose) This pose provides a great stretch for groin muscles, helps to strengthen and tone the muscles used for labor, and increases flexibility of knees and thighs.

How to do it: Sit on the mat with your back straight. You can also sit on a cushion or blanket to ease your hips. Roll shoulders away from ears and down the back. Draw the soles of the feet together and allow the knees to fall to either side. Interlace fingers around feet, cradling the toes. Draw heels as close to the body as feels comfortable. Ground yourself in this pose with the affirmation: "I am grounded, relaxed, and open, like a lotus blossom."

Earth Rooting Pose (or Mountain) This pose aligns the spine and can help encourage good posture. It brings a feeling of stability and groundedness, of standing firmly in your power. What could be sexier?

How to do it: Stand tall with legs hip-distance apart and feet parallel. Let arms hang alongside your body, with palms facing forward. Engage the muscles above the kneecaps, tucking the tailbone and directing it toward the earth. Lift your head to look straight ahead and draw the shoulders down the back. Inhale deeply, filling the lungs. Lift your toes and then spread them down into the mat. Feel your weight drop into your heels as if you were a tree, dropping roots deep into the earth. Take this moment to explore your connection with Mother Earth. Stand in this posture as long

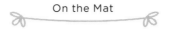

as it feels good, taking deep breaths, softening your gaze, and feeling the earth connection. Then continue by inhaling the arms up and overhead and exhaling them back down alongside the body. This posture is great to do at the beginning of each day. Ground yourself in the pose with the affirmation: "I am fully stable and supported by Mother Earth."

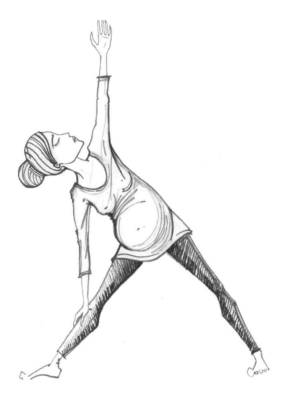

Sacred Triangle Pose: The downward-pointing triangle is used to represent water and earth—the female principle. Pythagoras considered the triangle sacred not only because of its perfect shape but also because he saw it as a symbol of universal fertility. We are powerful vessels for creation. That being said, many of us need to repattern beliefs we have about birth and our bodies. Think of your uterus as Pythagoras did: as the sacred fertile space that is the beginning of all life. That's something to glow about!

Some benefits of Sacred Triangle Pose include an increase in stamina; improved flexibility of the torso; strengthening of the ankles, feet, and legs; elongation of the spine; and a juicy opening of the hips.

How to do it: Start in Warrior II position: Start with legs together, feet turned out to a 45-degree angle, heels touching. Then slide the left leg back behind you, and bend the right knee deeply. Make sure you turn those right toes forward, parallel with the length of your mat. Left toes continue to point out 45 degrees. Inhale and stretch the arms out from the shoulders into a T-position, with palms facing down. From here move into Sacred Triangle: Hips pressing forward, hinge at the hip crease and reach front fingertips straight ahead. Rest the bottom arm on the shin or a yoga block, and raise your top arm toward the ceiling. Be careful not to rest your hand on your knee in this pose as the knee could hyperextend here with extra pressure. Gaze up at your top thumb. Feel the chest open in expansion. Hold for several breaths. Explore your connection with the divine with the affirmation: "I am a powerful creative force with sacred purpose."

Sound It Out!

Mantra, sound, and visualization can be used along with breathing techniques to take you out of your busy head and into your blooming womb. The connection between sound and opening is one worth exploring. As I mentioned earlier, when we relax the jaw and throat, the pelvic floor muscles relax. There is a hardwired connection between the mouth/throat and the vagina/pelvic floor muscles. Some of the pelvic floor muscles are sphincter muscles, or circular muscles that can open and close like a drawstring bag. The iris of your eye, which dilates and contracts, is an example of a sphincter muscle. Sphincter muscles surround the urethra, vagina, anus, and rectum, helping us to open and close these openings. We have similar circular sphincters in our digestive tract, mouth, and throat. All of these little round muscles are neurologically wired and coordinated with one another. So, what you do unto one, will happen to others as well. Learn to relax the mouth and throat to relax the pelvic floor, and you'll have a helpful tool during labor.

Bonus: Practicing making sounds also helps us become more relaxed when having sex—which is helpful both in terms of having more fun, and also from a fertility standpoint. The more open and relaxed you are during intimacy and high-level arousal, the better your chances at conceiving. The higher your arousal, the more your round ligaments contract. The round ligaments connect to the vulva and the uterus. At orgasm, the uterus contracts powerfully in a rhythm that is designed to suck semen up into the vagina like a straw, and back toward the cervical opening for conception. Essentially, when you orgasm, you increase your chances for fertilization. Now that's hot!

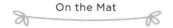

Sound turns off the thinking brain and helps amplify sensation. Good labor has a freeing sound, much like the primal erotic sounds of sex. Sounding helps to let down defenses and accelerate the labor. Sound is a gift, so get used to the power of your voice. Just like sexy sounds amplify your erotic experience and help you to reach orgasm, sexy sounds also help you to open up and expand to accommodate the passage of your baby. As the wise grandmother midwife Ina May Gaskin says, "The same energy that got the baby in will get the baby out." So those hot, sexy sounds will help you to open up. When you tense up and make high-pitched sounds, you constrict the throat and draw the pelvic floor muscles up and inward. So make sure you are keeping the voice low. I like to call it "pillow voice." Pillow voice is that tonal register you get when you wake up and suddenly start talking—or as you wind down for the night before bed. That sultry, raspy voice you have when you catch a cold? That's pillow voice. You want to stay in that range when you're doing yogic sound practice. Ready to try it? Great. Let's practice:

1. Find your way to a comfortable seated position. You may sit on the edge of a chair with your back nice and straight, on the floor in a cross-legged position, or on the floor and against a wall with your knees bent, feet pressing into the floor, legs spread open a bit wider than hip's distance.

2. Close your eyes. Take a long deep breath in, and on the exhale sigh audibly to release. Repeat this a few times and proceed with the next breath and sound, repeating each one at least three times before moving to the next set of sounds.

3. The next in-breath should be nice and full. On the exhale, relax your jaw and sound a nice *Ah* sound. Repeat three times.

4. Make the next in-breath full, once again. On the exhale find your inner animal and sound a deep *Oh*. Repeat three times.

5. Finally, take a deep breath in to prepare, and on the exhale make a low and sexy *Uhhh* sound. Repeat three times. (Or more—this one is especially fun, you can take it to the bedroom!)

Notice what happens in your pelvic floor over the course of this exercise. It should become more relaxed and open. Remember, when we're having sex, the sounds we make help the body to relax and ease into the sensations of ecstasy. The same rule is operating here.

These techniques will help you find your power in labor. Whether you are birthing at home, in the hospital, or at a birthing center, sound will help keep you in a place of primal power.

Affirmations for Inner Guidance

The word *center* reminds us to move into balance, to move toward the core, and to find stability. We want to surrender to what's happening in pregnancy and honor each aspect of the process. When we take the time to really connect with the miraculous gift that is unfolding, we are affirming the overflowing love that originates from within.

Your affirmations—positive declarative thoughts—should reflect positive intentions that speak to your experience and help shape your outlook on each day of your pregnancy.

My client Lucy had difficulty getting pregnant and would always start her sentences with "basically, I suck . . ." I could not understand why she chose that phrase for everything she had to say. When we got to the bottom of it all I discovered she thought she was constantly "making mistakes." I said to Lucy, "What if I told you your behaviors mirror what you think of yourself? You are prone to making mistakes because you believe that you will fail before you even get started. What if you began to affirm yourself with a different thought pattern, one that spoke to your greatness?"

We all have told ourselves things like *I'm stupid, I'll never be good enough,* and *I can't do it*—the list goes on, but you get the picture. These are declarative statements that affirm negative thought patterns. We do not want to give airtime to our negative thoughts; in fact, we want to do just the opposite. It's the negative voice that plays over and over like a broken record that got you to stop believing in yourself in the first place. I'm here to take the needle off the record and flip the focus to the positive. Instead of focusing on what you don't want, here in the first trimester and throughout your Mama Glow pregnancy you will focus on what you *do* want. What you think about you bring about, so think positively. If you've never said an affirmation, that's fine. You're learning to expand the arsenal of tools you have to help you turn up the glow volume.

Here are some basic guidelines for creating a positive affirmation:

• Choose an area to focus on in your life.

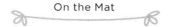

- Make a positive declarative statement, based in the present. "I am relaxed and calm" rather than "I have no stress."

- Affirmations should be personal, as they are tools for manifestation. Always use the word *I*.

- Affirmations should be specific. "I am confident" is nice, but "I am confident in my body's ability to birth my baby" is going to be more effective because it's specific.

- Just like with magic, you have to believe it's true or possible for your affirmation to really take hold and make a difference. Examples of affirmations:

  - I am a strong and wise woman; I trust the infinite wisdom of my body in this process.

  - My inner wisdom is guiding me now.

  - I am now an open channel for creative energy.

  - I now feel deep inner peace and serenity.

  - I am beautiful, complete, and abundant with life.

  - I am taking the best care of myself and my baby.

One of my favorite birthing affirmations comes from Harriette Hartigan's *Of Nature and Birth*. In this video, the images of blooming flowers are set to this mantra: "I am opening up in sweet surrender to this beautiful baby in my womb."

Take a moment to come up with some affirmations that make sense for you. If you have self-doubt or aren't used to affirming yourself, this is a great exercise to boost confidence and begin to acknowledge your powerful inner resources. Daily affirmations were a huge part of my labor and birth, and I continue to use them to bring about inner peace and calm. I would say, "Many women before me have done this. I am fully equipped with all I need to have my baby." I offer this example to all my clients so they know they aren't alone—that they are part of a continuum of women who have all given birth really helps to change the perspective. I'm glad you will be taking these tools with you. Find great guided affirmations and meditations on my website www.mamaglow.com.

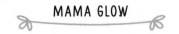

Mama Glow Checklist:

- ☐ Purchase mat, blocks, bolster, and other accessories for your yoga practice.
- ☐ Download guided meditations and affirmations.
- ☐ Write your own affirmations and practice daily.

You got your Om on, grounding yourself in postures, exploring some affirmations, and even playing with sound. You're developing a practice that you can continue for the duration of pregnancy and into postpartum. Next we'll dive into your sacred anatomy and divine femininity.

CHAPTER 8

IN YOUR LIFE

Sacred Anatomy

I'd like to take a moment to speak about the use of words. In studying sacred anatomy and Hindu texts I came across a beautiful word to describe the female genitalia: *yoni.* The word *yoni* describes the downward-pointing triangle that symbolizes the womb. It speaks to the sacredness of this part of the body. Each letter of the word in Sanskrit has an esoteric meaning defining the innermost content of the word itself (while the word is pronounced *yo-nee*, the Sanskrit word is written as *yoin*):

Y: The animating principle, the heart, the true self, union
O: Preservation, brightness
I: Love, desire, consciousness, to shine, to pervade pain and sorrow
N: Lotus, motherhood, menstrual cycle, nakedness, emptiness, pearl

The female sacred anatomy is a multifunctional and integrated system designed to make babies and to experience pleasure and attachment. The words we use have powerful meaning, so we should feel good about them. The word *vagina* comes from Latin, meaning "sheath," as to a sword. In other words, a container for a man's "sword," or penis. It's not exactly empowering language to use to describe these sacred organs! Many women lack connection with their body parts, referring to their most intimate parts as "down there." We expect our sexual partners to know exactly how to navigate our intimate topography, and yet oftentimes we don't have a sense of what pleasures us. How can you feel good about birth when you're not relating to your own sacred anatomy? This disconnected behavior reflects a warped cultural view of the female body. We've had a lot of negative conditioning about our body parts, which stretches far beyond the scope of this book. But we are here to invoke the divine within our bodies. We have to remember that we are holy. Nothing is more sacred than the creative process. Passive engagement with our bodies means we are not living to our fullest pleasure potential. We must not only respect but also *reclaim* our bodies.

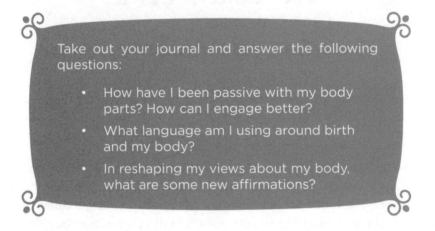

Take out your journal and answer the following questions:

- How have I been passive with my body parts? How can I engage better?

- What language am I using around birth and my body?

- In reshaping my views about my body, what are some new affirmations?

Ode to My Belly and Thighs

Pregnancy is an opportunity to finally address any neuroses we have about our bodies. We are constantly hearing through cultural messaging that we are not enough. We reaffirm that messaging every day when we roll our eyes at the circumference of our thighs and suck in our bellies to fit into skinny jeans.

I admire my dear friend Doutzen Kroes, a Victoria's Secret supermodel and new haute mama, for her commitment to living the Mama Glow lifestyle and to not perpetuating the negative view of the female body. At a conference for the CFDA, a fashion institution, Doutzen publicly spoke out against the ultra-small sample sizes that are the industry standard. An avid yogini who loves boxing, jump rope, and green juice, Doutzen enjoys working out and Eating well to stay healthy. Everybody is demanding the models fit into a 33-inch-hip sample size. As a reference point, a teenage boy has a 32-inch hip! Do we really want to celebrate an ideal

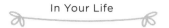

of young women that look like prepubescent boys? Doutzen remains one of the highest-paid supermodels in the industry and with the birth of her new baby boy she snapped right back into shape in a healthy way through rest, good diet, and breastfeeding. "I love my body and I made the choice to be healthy. And I have joy in what I do because I'm not hungry all the time." Doutzen is a Mama Glow Icon not only because she embodies the lifestyle principles but also because she stands fiercely for what she believes and is living her life on her own terms.

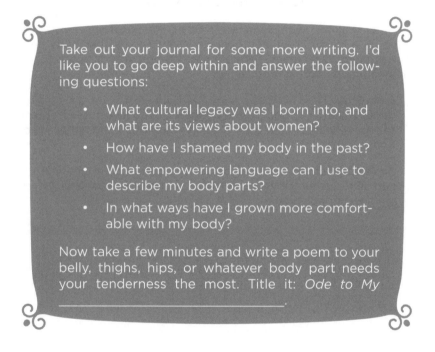

Take out your journal for some more writing. I'd like you to go deep within and answer the following questions:

- What cultural legacy was I born into, and what are its views about women?
- How have I shamed my body in the past?
- What empowering language can I use to describe my body parts?
- In what ways have I grown more comfortable with my body?

Now take a few minutes and write a poem to your belly, thighs, hips, or whatever body part needs your tenderness the most. Title it: *Ode to My* _____.

Feeling secure and confident in your body is an ongoing process. During this first trimester, we are all coming to a place of healing in our lives.

Here are some affirmations for self-love:

- Today, I honor my body. I love myself, and I treat myself with respect.
- I listen only to my own inner wisdom and let it guide my every thought and action.
- Today I celebrate my belly, hips, and thighs as a reminder of my divine femininity.

To really operate from a place of total power you have to embody your divinity, your holy glow. Harness that inner power. Not only is it your birthright, honey, it's your responsibility. Next stop: Second Trimester. You're a third of the way there! As your glow pilot, I want you to know that we're moving into the glow zone, and pretty soon you'll be riding on cruise control.

Glow Tips for Self-Love

Rebecca Walker, writer, luminary, mother, and author of *Baby Love* and *Black Cool,* is a Mama Glow Icon because she embraces her body and celebrates her miraculous curves. Rebecca has two practical glow tips for loving your changing body during pregnancy.

- *Love Gaze.* Sit in front of a mirror without clothes on and take a good look at your body's every contour. Send love and acceptance to your reflection. Take your favorite oil or lotion and lather your body.

- *Be Photographed.* Whether by your partner or a professional, allow yourself to embrace your sensuality, suppleness, and femininity. Enjoy this glorious time.

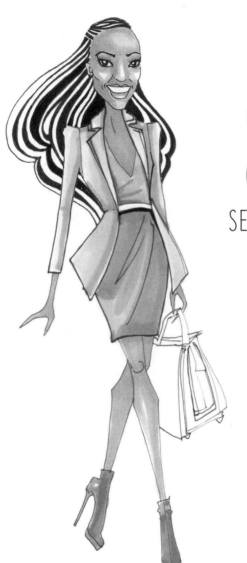

part III

GET YOUR GLOW ON!

SECOND TRIMESTER
(WEEKS 14–28)

CHAPTER 9

A BUN IN THE OVEN

Now You're Cookin'

I remember the burst of energy I felt when I entered into my second trimester. It was the glow zone. I felt like I could do anything, including things I had no business doing—like carrying my groceries up three flights of stairs or attending the launch of a swanky New York nightclub. Nearly nine years ago the mayor of New York passed a law that prohibited smoking in nightclubs and restaurants, which was huge! I could finally go with my boyfriend to some of the fabulous events we were invited to. The very evening the law passed we got all dressed up to go to an event. I was worried that I would be the only pregnant goddess in the building. To my delight, it turned out I wasn't the only one: there were five other gorgeous mamas getting down on the dance floor, too!

In the second trimester, we're really cooking! Pregnancy is a psychological journey as well as a biological one. During the second trimester, you may feel less tired and more up to the challenge of preparing a home for your baby. Strike while the iron is hot! Check into childbirth education classes. Find a health-care provider for your baby. Focus on your commitment to healthy lifestyle choices that will give your baby the best start. Here in Part III, we are exploring changes in body and mind, common discomforts, and more food, yoga, and beauty solutions.

A Glance at Baby's Development in the Second Trimester

- *Week 16:* Tiny bones are forming in the ears; eyebrows, lashes, and hair are starting to fill in.
- *Week 18:* Baby has become mobile: yawning, kicking, punching, rolling and twisting, hiccupping, sucking, and swallowing.
- *Week 20:* Baby is gulping down amniotic fluid, practicing swallowing; his or her taste buds are working.
- *Week 22:* Baby is sleeping 12 to 14 hours per day.
- *Week 24:* Baby is packing on the fat! Skin is becoming opaque; small capillaries are giving the skin pigment.
- *Week 26:* Baby's immune system is soaking up antibodies and his or her eyes are forming, too.

Mama's Development in the Second Trimester

You're rocking and rolling my friend. You may have more energy than you did in the first three months. Hopefully you're starting to feel like you're glowing! If you were experiencing any morning sickness, by now it's a thing of the past. Your mood swings may lessen, especially if you are eating glow foods. This will be a good time to tackle many tasks necessary to get ready for your baby. You'll start to gain more weight this trimester, adding as much as three pounds a month for the rest of your pregnancy. This means you may need to start wearing maternity clothes. But that doesn't mean that fashion goes out the door, thank goodness. There are

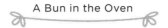

many designers who have considered the stylish mama's needs. Your breasts may not be as tender as they were in the first trimester, but they will continue to grow and prepare for breastfeeding, aided by enlarged milk glands and deposits of fat. You may also notice that the skin on and around your nipples will darken, and you might have small bumps around the nipples themselves. These bumps are called Montgomery glands, which will begin to secrete an oily substance to keep your nipples supple and prepare them for breastfeeding. Speaking of nipples, you may notice a yellowish fluid, called colostrum, starting to leak out of your breasts. Don't be alarmed—it's totally normal. Also normal will be increased sensitivity to the sun, meaning you might burn more easily. Be sure to protect yourself more than usual. Finally, you may see a dark line, the *linea nigra*, form down the middle of your belly from your navel to your pubic hair.

Top Three Second-Trimester Challenges

Sleeplessness

Nearly all pregnant women have some challenge with sleep at one point or another. The same pregnancy hormone that causes fatigue during the day—progesterone—can disrupt your sleep cycle at night. This may include trouble falling asleep, waking up during the night, trouble falling back to sleep, and sleep that just isn't restful.

A number of problems can contribute to your sleeplessness during pregnancy, including:

- Difficulty finding a comfortable position for sleeping with the increasing size of your belly.

- Awaking several times throughout the night to pee.

- Anxiety and stress.

- Leg cramps, hemorrhoids, and round ligament pain in your hip flexor region.

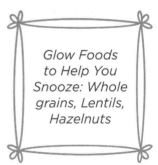

Glow Foods to Help You Snooze: Whole grains, Lentils, Hazelnuts

Here's what you can do:

- Breathe deep. Practice your deep breathing or simply close your eyes and imagine a peaceful scene while taking long deep breaths.

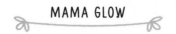

This will relax your nervous system and set you up for some good sleep.

- Take naps when inspired. Nap when possible during the day. This can help you avoid getting too tired, especially if you have a hard time getting restful sleep at night.

- Avoid sleeping flat on your back. This position puts the full weight of your uterus on your back and on the vena cava, the vein that carries blood between your lower body and your heart. Sleeping on your back can also increase your chances of getting backaches and can aggravate digestive problems, heartburn, and hemorrhoids. Try to get used to sleeping on your side, particularly on your left side as this maximizes blood flow to your baby. This position can improve your circulation and help reduce any swelling in your feet.

- Have a pillow party. Tuck one pillow between your legs, then another between your feet so your hips are stacked. Use more pillows to support your back and abdomen. If you've been experiencing heartburn or shortness of breath during pregnancy, use pillows to prop up your upper body while you sleep.

- Make your room comfortable. I only do two things in my bed. Sleeping is one of them; you can guess the other! Use your bed only for sleeping and intimacy. When you start inviting other activities, like surfing the web, it sends a signal to your mind that it's not time to sleep. Make sure the room is at a comfortable temperature. Play some relaxing or natural sounds to help make you sleepy. If you like, open a window so you have access to fresh air.

- Go to bed earlier. You may need to turn in sooner during the second trimester, especially if you find yourself waking up several times during the night. I couldn't stay up past 9 P.M. when I was pregnant, but I had girlfriends who were up watching Conan at this stage because they couldn't get cozy. Go to bed when you feel tired. Don't impose a bedtime that doesn't feel right, but listen to your body's signals.

- Avoid getting up during the night. Try not to drink anything for two or three hours before bedtime. This will reduce the number of times you need to get up for a trip to the toilet. If nighttime heartburn is

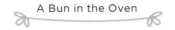

kicking your butt, eat your last meal of the day several hours before lying down to go to sleep. To prevent nighttime leg cramps, gently stretch your legs and take a calcium/magnesium supplement. It will help eliminate cramps and has the added bonus of sending you soundly to sleep.

- Move your body, girl. Yes, I know you're pregnant. That doesn't mean you can't exercise. At this stage, it's important to get at least 2½ hours of aerobic exercise every week. This means 30 minutes of aerobic exercise on most days. Moderate exercise, like Mama Glow yoga or walking, regulates your circadian rhythm and can help you get a better night's sleep. Always be sure to find out from your health-care provider what exercises are safe for you and how long you can maintain your exercise program.

Reflux/Indigestion/Heartburn

By now you may be fairly well acquainted with the feelings of indigestion, heartburn, and acid reflux. I remember the first time I realized I could no longer eat the local Punjabi dal and rice because the onions gave me a mean case of heartburn. It was so bad that I thought I'd developed a heart condition! During pregnancy, your hormones relax the muscles in your digestive tract, including the valve in the esophagus. This allows stomach acids to more easily seep back up the esophagus, especially when you're lying down. Heartburn can be worse in the second and third trimesters, when your growing uterus presses on your stomach, sometimes pushing food back up into the esophagus.

Some additional causes of reflux and heartburn include:

- The muscles that push food from your esophagus into your stomach are more relaxed.

- The muscles that contract to digest food in your stomach are also more relaxed, which slows down your digestion—meaning there is more food in your stomach for longer periods of time.

- Other changes to the stomach can lead to indigestion, which can make you feel very full, bloated, and gassy.

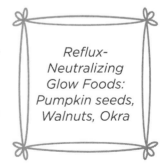

Reflux-Neutralizing Glow Foods: Pumpkin seeds, Walnuts, Okra

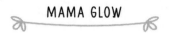
- As your uterus expands, it compresses your stomach and other digestive organs, making you feel fuller faster.

Here's what you can do:

- Eat smaller meals. Eat five or six small meals a day instead of eating three larger meals. Because of the increased compression of your stomach, smaller meals will feel better. Snacks are key, so load up on fiber-rich glow foods to keep you moving.

- Drink less while eating. Avoid drinking with your meals. Instead, drink your fluids—particularly water and coconut water—between meals.

- Avoid foods that trigger heartburn. Avoid spicy, greasy, or fatty foods, as well as onions, garlic, citrus, tomatoes, mustard, chocolate, and, of course, caffeine.

- Take glutamine. The digestive tract uses glutamine as a fuel source and for self-healing of stomach ulcers, reflux, irritable bowel syndrome, and ulcerative bowel diseases. Begin with 8 g daily for a trial period of four weeks to see how your body responds.

- Take your probiotics. Probiotic remedies include Lactobacillus acidophilus and bifidus. Although not a cure in themselves, these friendly bacteria are an important addition to any protocol for the gut. Acidophilus is best taken at bedtime. Some women only tolerate the Lactobacillus acidophilus, without the bifidus.

- Try slippery elm bark. Slippery elm bark has demulcent properties, meaning it has a slimy coating effect, and has long been a folk remedy for heartburn and ulcers. It can be used in large amounts without harm. Drink as tea, chew on the bark, or take in capsule form, starting with 2 to 4 capsules three times daily for a trial period of three weeks. To make a tea, simmer 1 teaspoon of slippery elm bark in 2 cups of water for 20 minutes and strain. You can get slippery elm tea at your natural foods store or online.

- Take zinc. Zinc increases the healing of the gut lining and can prevent future damage to the stomach lining. Take 50 mg daily.

- Take EFAs—evening primrose, borage, or flaxseed oils. These oils increase the levels of prostaglandin E2 series, which promotes healing and repair. Take up to 1,000 mg of any one of these oils—or

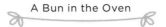

1,000 mg of a combination of all three—three times a day for a trial period of four weeks. Prostaglandins ripen the cervix, preparing you for delivery—which is great when you are in the home stretch, but you don't want to overdo it at this point! Consider including flaxseed oil in your combination, as it is an excellent source of linoleic acid, an essential fatty acid. Low dietary intake of linoleic acid has been associated with duodenal ulcers. You may want to use ground flaxseed rather than the oil, as the mucous portion of the flaxseed buffers excess acid, which makes it ideal for inflammation in the stomach and throughout the gastrointestinal tract. Grind seeds daily or buy ground flaxseed products with enhanced shelf life and store in the refrigerator.

> **Glow Tip:** Linoleic acid is also found in pumpkin seeds, tofu, walnuts, safflower oil, sunflowers seeds and oil, and sesame seeds and oil. Use 2 to 3 teaspoons in smoothies or protein drinks, or on salads and vegetables.

Sluggish Bowels/Constipation

What's the scoop on your poop? Not much happening? A normal transit time for waste to make it through your body is 12 to 18 hours. Yet the average American stool transit time is 72 hours. Why? Because our diet doesn't contain the fiber or water we need to get things moving. We absorb 20 liters of water per day just through our colon alone. Constipation is a very common experience for pregnant women, to boot. One reason is an increase in the hormone progesterone, which relaxes smooth muscles throughout the body, including the digestive tract. Food passes through the intestines more slowly. This, along with the pressure of your growing uterus on your rectum, makes it hard for a girl to handle her business in the bathroom. Iron supplements, particularly in high doses, can make constipation even worse.

Here's what you can do about constipation:

- Eat high-fiber foods. Include foods such as whole grains, brown rice, beans, and fresh fruits in the early part of the day and lots of green veggies all day long. Adding a couple of tablespoons of ground flax or chia seeds to your smoothie in the morning will also make a difference.

- Drink plenty of water. At least eight glasses a day. A glass of stone-fruit juice like plum or prune juice every day can also be helpful. Some people find that drinking warm water with lemon right after waking up helps get things moving (as you'll remember, it's part of the prepregnancy detox I recommended in Chapter 2).

- Exercise regularly. Walking, yoga, swimming, and dancing can all help ease constipation and leave you feeling more fit, healthy, and relieved.

- Make time for the toilet. Your bowels are most likely to be active after meals, so make time to use the bathroom after you eat. Listen to your body. Never put off going to the bathroom when you feel the urge.

- Cut back on iron. Many prenatal multivitamins contain a large dose of iron. Ask your health-care provider about switching to a supplement with less iron. In its place, try stinging nettles—a powerful herb that's loaded with iron that's easy to assimilate. Drink it as a tea to help loosen things up.

- Take calcium and magnesium. Magnesium is the headliner mineral activating over 350 different processes including digestion, muscle function, energy production, bone formation, enzyme function, activation of B vitamins, and more. It also helps with constipation. Take it at night in combination with calcium, which will relax you for bedtime and deliver a stool promptly upon waking!

Glow Foods for Good Poop: Pears, Kale, Brazil nuts

From Home Births to Hospitals:
Where, How, and Who Will Deliver?

Choosing *where*, *how*, and *who* will deliver your baby are three of the most important decisions you will make. These are very personal choices; you should know your options and do what resonates best with you and your partner.

Where: Home Birth, Birth Center, or Hospital?

When I first learned I was pregnant I had no idea where to go for care. I did what any first-time mom-to-be with no clue would do—I pulled out the Yellow Pages! (I wasn't as internet savvy back then.) I called around only to find there were enormous waiting lists for practitioners, and I was looking at a three- to five-month wait for some of the MDs. I knew I wanted a more natural route, but I wasn't quite sure how to go about it, or even where to go. My son's father and I started off at a maternity care center connected with Columbia University, but it didn't feel quite right. Even though my caretaker was a wise midwife, something about the place itself—the staff and protocol—didn't sit well with us. Then we discovered there was a childbearing center about nine blocks away from our apartment—even with the same house number as our place, 222. I was intrigued by this place, which was sandwiched between a nightclub and a secondhand/vintage clothing shop. At this point I was going into 28 weeks, just at their cut-off for taking new birth clients. I attended an informational session and fell in love with the practice. What I loved about the birth center were the kind and gentle midwives. I felt totally at home, my visits weren't rushed, and I had total access to my files. The room where I delivered had a huge Jacuzzi, low lighting, a queen-sized bed that fit me and my partner, and a large bathroom. It was decorated like a home and made me feel totally comfortable.

If my living conditions at the time were different, I would have explored having a home birth. If you decide to brave it out at home, there are a few things you should know. First and foremost, most doctors will not attend home births because of malpractice insurance constraints. You should, however, be able to find a nurse midwife to attend your home birth. Home births have a few perks. You're in your own familiar environment, so there is a feeling of safety, which helps labor progress. Unlike a hospital setting, there aren't a bunch of other ladies delivering at the same time—so you have the full attention of your midwife. You can move around freely and eat, as you are not being continuously monitored by machines. If you give birth at home, I would consider having an inflatable birthing pool to labor in. My home birth clients swear by water birth, as water has an analgesic effect on the body and can help a laboring mom ease her way into motherhood. I spent much of my time laboring in water myself.

Midwives are very skilled with comfort measures and are known to be very patient with the birth process—which can help the laboring mother feel safe and empowered in her labor. The midwife will bring her superhero toolbox, including a Doppler, stethoscope, scalpel, hemostat, first-aid kit, and oxygen. Hiring a labor-support coach, also known as a doula, as well as having a close friend there with you when you move into active labor, is a great way to ensure you feel constant support when you need it most.

If you prefer to work with a doctor, you will most likely deliver in a hospital, though some will deliver in birthing centers like the one I used. If your doctor practices at a fixed location, you may not have much of a choice when it comes to the "where" aspect of your delivery. If you want to deliver somewhere more chill, where it feels like you're at home rather than in an episode of *Grey's Anatomy*, then aim for a birth center. Birthing centers come in two different types. You have your freestanding centers, which is as it sounds: a building not directly connected to a hospital. Then you have your hospital birth center, which is a separate, more homey-feeling space within the hospital itself. The latter option may be a good choice for someone who wants the security of being in a hospital and having doctors nearby, minus the weird lighting and smells.

At a freestanding birth center there is virtually no intervention—meaning you give birth without the assistance of drugs or anything that would modulate the natural process. In a birth center within a hospital, medical interventions like induction and epidural anesthesia are possible but less likely than if you were birthing within the hospital itself. You will also be able to make more decisions about your delivery as needed. If you want to switch positions, take a shower, labor in the tub, or eat and drink, you can. After your baby arrives, you are also discharged much earlier than you would be if you were in the hospital. I remember walking out the door six hours after I delivered my son in total awe that six hours prior he was inside of me. That said, birth centers are not equipped to deal with sudden emergencies the way hospitals are, so if (God forbid) there were a complication, you would need to be transported to the nearest hospital.

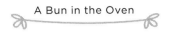
How: Birth *Au Naturel* or Pain Management?

When we signed on at the birth center, I knew that I was mentally and emotionally preparing myself for the most intense and pivotal experience of my life. I
also knew that the birth center would not offer pain management through drugs.
There wasn't anything on site, even if I had wanted it. When a mama says she had
a "natural birth," that usually means a vaginal birth where little or no drugs/inter-
ventions were involved. While many of my clients are aiming for natural birth, I
like to go one better and call it "supernatural birth." What I mean by *supernatural*
is an unobstructed and totally supported birth where a laboring mother's innate
wisdom is guiding the process—including the production of chemicals that make
the process more pleasurable and less painful. I took the natural route and found
that my body governed the process better than any man-made drug could. I had
a swift and fairly easy labor that I am certain would have been prolonged had I
been in a different setting with pain medications available to me. If you want to
feel all the sensations of your labor, the idea of natural birth may float your boat. I
have some moms who are very clear in the beginning that pain is a threshold that
they cannot cross alone, however, so we open the conversation about pain management and find their comfort zone. I recommend getting familiar with the Alex-
ander technique—which is a simple and practical method for improving ease and
freedom of movement, balance, and flexibility, and descent of the baby through
the sacred passageway—and taking childbirth classes. You'll want to be prepped
on the physiology of labor and equipped with some breathing techniques. You'll
also want to familiarize yourself with various effective coping techniques for labor
that don't involve drugs. Some of these include essential oils, acupressure, counterpressure, deep breathing, visualization, and water. Think about what natural
birth means to you. What it meant for me was that I chose to stay consciously connected to the divine surge moving through me—that my baby and I stayed in total
sync in the process of labor.

Over 60 percent of women who deliver in hospitals ultimately choose epidural
anesthesia, which is injected in the epidural shaft around the spinal cord. It takes
the edge off the pain for laboring moms, meaning there is little awareness of what
is happening below the beltline. Some moms opt for the epi so they can get some
good rest and be strong for the transition, or pushing, phase.

I once attended a birth that started off with 30 hours of intense contractions,
and the mommy just wasn't getting comfortable at home. Once we arrived at the
hospital they checked her cervix to find that she was three centimeters dilated,

which she found extremely discouraging considering she had labored so long at home. At that point she was faced with a decision, be admitted to the hospital where she could have an epidural and relax, or go back home and manage the discomfort naturally. The choice for her was very clear: epidural and rest. We worked through the guilt she had around changing her mind, but I assured her to trust her decision and allow her body to rest so she would have energy to push out her baby. She got comfortable in the room, put on her iPod and slept. Her labor actually kicked into high gear once she was comfortable, and three hours later she was pushing and delivered a healthy baby girl. That was a beautiful example of the compassionate use and power of an epidural.

Since for the most part you have to stay in bed once it's administered, having an epidural makes it harder to move into new positions to help move your baby down into the sacred passageway (birth canal). Hormone production also halts, and the lack of sensation can prolong the pushing phase. Other possible side effects to an epidural include:

- Sudden drop in blood pressure. For this reason your blood pressure will be routinely checked to make sure there is adequate blood flow to your baby. If your blood pressure drops you may need to be treated with IV fluids, medications, and oxygen.

- Severe headache. This pain is often caused by leakage of spinal fluid. Less than 1 percent of women experience this side effect, but it's worth knowing about.

- Other miscellaneous effects. These may include shivering, ringing of the ears, backache, soreness where the needle is inserted, nausea, and difficulty urinating.

Talk to your practitioner about alternatives to having an epidural. Some moms opt for morphine, Stadol, or Demerol.

Who: OB or Midwife?

If you have a strong relationship with your OB/GYN, you may choose to transition that relationship into the pregnancy. This familiar face will be the best choice for you if you have certain known complications or risks. That said, if you want a little more personalized attention and a level of flexibility, you don't have to feel like you're cheating on your OB/GYN to play the field and find a midwife. You may just fall in love and fall into good hands. A certified nurse midwife (CNM) has a nursing degree, extra training in monitoring pregnancy and delivering babies, and tends to have a little more time to spend with patients during prenatal visits and the labor process. Some midwives even do home prenatal visits and house calls postpartum—now that's what I call customer service! Midwives are in the little-to-no-intervention camp, so for a low-risk pregnancy this is a well-aligned choice.

The question of doctor or midwife really comes down to whom you feel most comfortable with—who you like and trust. This is your party! You can invite whomever you want to. Just make sure you dig your practitioner. He or she will be an integral part of your birth team—and your world—for the rest of your pregnancy.

Gestational Diabetes

Diabetes is not an easy-breezy subject. It means you have abnormally high levels of sugar in your blood, which can be dangerous to you *and* your baby.

When you eat, your digestive system breaks down most of your food into glucose. The glucose enters your bloodstream and then, with the help of insulin, is absorbed as fuel by your cells. If, however, your body doesn't produce enough insulin—or your cells have a problem responding to it—that glucose remains in your blood instead of being converted to energy by your cells. The result is unusual fatigue (because the cells are being starved of energy), increased or rapid weight gain, and increased blood pressure, related to high levels of insulin in the bloodstream.

When you're pregnant, hormonal changes can make your cells less responsive to insulin—meaning they need more of it. For most moms-to-be, this isn't a problem: when the body needs additional insulin, the pancreas dutifully secretes it. But if your pancreas can't keep up with the increased insulin demand, your blood glucose levels rise too high. The result is gestational diabetes.

Insulin is a hormone which is excreted by the pancreas and allows glucose to pass into cells to be utilized as fuel. Simple sugars are rapidly absorbed by the small intestine, and once they're flowing into the bloodstream, the brain signals the pancreas to secrete insulin. Elevated insulin causes the body to burn sugar and store fat. Any fat contained in the meal as well as fat in the tissues is being stored when you eat a meal including processed foods and simple sugars. Insulin acts as the cell's gatekeeper for blood sugar. Regular exercise burns blood sugar and fat, keeps the insulin levels low, and empties the muscles of stored glucose.

When you have a cookie, for instance, your blood is flooded with sugars. The pancreas reacts by secreting lots of insulin. You now have high insulin and high blood sugar, which your body perceives as "code red" and a potential threat to your health. Your body wants to dump the sugar ASAP, so it burns sugar but not fat. Fat then gets stored. This is how mamas with gestational diabetes gain weight; and their little ones are often bigger in size as well. If you are managing gestational diabetes you should be working closely with a nutritionist, preferably a holistic-oriented one, who will address the underlying causes concerning diet and lifestyle.

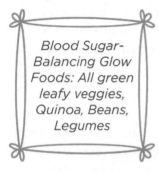

Blood Sugar-Balancing Glow Foods: All green leafy veggies, Quinoa, Beans, Legumes

The good news is you have some control over this condition. My friend Suzie, a prominent Ashtanga yoga practitioner and children's yoga instructor, was diagnosed with gestational diabetes during her fifth month of pregnancy. She was shocked, because she is such a healthy eater. Suzie kicked into high gear, reorienting her diet toward low-glycemic foods. She cut out rice and other starches, as well as fruit and dairy. When she returned to her doctor a few weeks later, she had completely reversed the condition.

Tips for managing gestational diabetes:

- Don't skip meals. Be consistent about when you eat meals and the amount of food you eat at each one. Your blood sugar will remain more stable if your food is distributed evenly throughout the day—and consistently from day to day.

- Eat a good breakfast. Your blood glucose levels are the most erratic in the morning. To keep your levels in a healthy range, you must limit carbohydrates (breads, cereals, and fruits) and boost your protein (almond butter, Brazil nuts, and walnuts). Avoid fruit, dried fruit, and fruit juice altogether.

- Boost your fiber. Include high-fiber foods in your diet throughout the day, including leafy green veggies, whole grains, hot cereals, and dried peas, beans, and legumes. These foods are broken down and absorbed more slowly than simple carbohydrates, which help keep your blood sugar levels in check after meals.

The second trimester is a wonderful time to check in with yourself and assess where you are on the glow spectrum. Are you ready to kick it up a notch? In Chapter 10, In the Kitchen, you will delve into conscious meal prep and glow grazing, preparing the best foods for you right now with total intention.

IN THE KITCHEN

Conscious Cooking and Eating for the Glow

You've heard the phrase "barefoot and pregnant," right? Well, something about shuffling around the kitchen barefoot grounded me during my pregnancy. Cooking was such a delight, and since my kitchen was out of commission during my pregnancy I would weasel my way into any nice kitchen I could find, just to fulfill my urge to bang pots and pans and make beautiful, tasty food. Needless to say, I was welcomed with open arms into many homes to satisfy my deep urge to cook.

Cooking should be a joyous process and not a burden. If you are feeling the pressure of meal preparation at this point in your pregnancy, don't be afraid to call upon your sister circle of women friends, your family members, and your beloved for help. If you have a husband or partner, encourage them to participate in shopping, prepping, and cooking. Cooking is alchemy, after all. When food enters your body it transforms your blood, your thoughts, your feelings—and becomes your actions. Since your body is your home, the energy you put into it through the food you eat is very important.

It's great to eat at restaurants. I love it myself, as I live in one of the most sophisticated cities on the planet when it comes to food. You can get anything you want in New York, from 5-star dining to food trucks. There is something tasty for your every whim. And yet, there's something very intimate about preparing your own food that, for me, makes it superior to eating out. In many restaurants, food is prepared in kitchens where line chefs are in a frenzy trying to get everyone's meals finished and out to the dining room. The cooks are overworked and underpaid, and the environment can sometimes border on the abusive. There isn't much love and peaceful energy going into preparing the food. Often the conditions in industrial and commercial kitchens are less than optimal for high-quality, clean food. So during this important time, I suggest you make food at home—developing a visceral connection to what you are eating.

The act of preparing food is one of love. It's a meditation. Feeding yourself and others is one of the most primal experiences. It's the act of feeding that bonds mother and baby. Part of the reason so many of us don't eat as well as we'd like—beyond the excuses we make—is that we don't believe we really deserve to sit down and have a home-cooked meal. Who has the time? There's so much else we could be doing. So instead, we nosh on snacks and cut corners with nutrition. Then we blame ourselves for eating poorly when we didn't set the tone by properly preparing a nutritious meal. I have a lovely client who, instead of cooking a proper meal for herself, would always opt for tortilla chips, hummus, and a bowl of edamame. I had to help her get to the bottom of why she was always taking shortcuts when it came to her well-being and get her to value *herself* as much as her work, so that cooking became a priority.

Before you prepare to cook, take a deep breath. Take the moment to set an intention and get your mind focused on the food before you begin. I play music like disco or love ballads while I am cooking. I even get my son involved in the process, so it's a pleasant family affair. He joins me to shop for ingredients, and I provide him with age-appropriate activities in the kitchen.

Here are some guidelines to successful cooking:

- Get equipped. As I said in Chapter 6, it's incredibly important to have the right equipment on hand. Think proper knives, pots, pans, cutting boards, blender, and food processor—the whole nine yards.

- Experiment. Try new things—new cooking techniques and new ingredients.

- Cook once, eat twice. To make the best use of your cooking time, prepare more food than you need so you can extend the meal into your week. This works especially well with grains and soup.

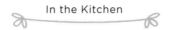

- Keep it simple. Keep your ingredient lists to a minimum until you get comfortable in the kitchen. Most of the recipes you'll find in this book are very simple.

- Get sassy with spices. Herbs and spices will help bring out the natural flavor in your food. They also connect us to ancestral flavors, reminding us of foods connected to us culturally.

Mindful Cooking Principles

Preparing food is a ritual, and I'd love for you to establish rituals that become a part of your lifestyle. My busy moms have few creative outlets, so I often give them a cooking assignment to allow their creativity to shine through. Slow-cooking recipes are a great way to calm the mind and enter a more meditative state. One of my dear friends and mentors Jill Wodnick has a saying she uses when folks stress her out: she tells them to "go stir some soup!" I now use it when talking to my wound-up moms when they are moving faster than a New York minute.

Food Combining: *Food combining* means designing your diet to accommodate proper digestion, utilization, and assimilation of nutrients. It is a basic component of optimal nutrition because it allows the body to digest and utilize the nutrients in our foods to their full extent. The discomforts of indigestion are so common today they're almost considered normal. The fact that over $2 billion is spent each year on antacids is proof enough. Different foods require different digestive enzymes—some acid, some alkaline. Protein foods require a highly acidic environment for digestion, while carbohydrates (starches, fruits, and sugars) and fats require a more alkaline medium. Any time two or more foods are eaten at the same time, and those foods require opposite conditions for digestion, the digestive process is compromised. When starches and proteins are combined, their stimulation of the digestive juices generates a conflicting response and produces an environment that does not digest either very well. This situation often leads to indigestion, bloating, gas, abdominal discomfort, and poor absorption of nutrients. Be conscious about which foods you are pairing together. For more information on food pairing, I recommend *The Complete Book of Food Combining: A New Approach to the Hay Diet and Healthy Eating,* by Jan and Inge Dries. Take the time to learn the basics.

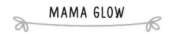
The Importance of Gratitude—and Attitude: Your attitude in the kitchen is extremely important. Coming from a place of gratitude, feeling thankful for what you have and sharing what you have with others, will not only make you feel good, it will make your *food* good. It's that extra ingredient—the love factor—that your grandmother always added to her cookies. Play music you love while you cook, think positive thoughts, and let your family get involved in the cooking process.

The Importance of Foundation and Balance: Having a strong foundation in nutrition and balanced eating is key to living a healthy lifestyle. One must develop an understanding of what foods to eat and how they are processed in your body. Use yourself as an experiment.

Intuitive Cooking: Allow your creativity to flow in the kitchen. It's not all about recipes; it's about sensing what is right for you, listening to your inner voice, your palate, and your mood. Try preparing something without a recipe next time and see what happens. If you engage your senses when eating, you will develop the ability to discern what ingredients are in a dish. In my family my grandmother and mother both have this ability. They can be in a restaurant and experience a meal, then deconstruct the flavors and re-create something similar and better at home. Cooking from intuition means you won't need to follow so many steps, making cooking less mechanical and more artful—a true celebration of food.

The Power of Your Intention: When you set out to prepare a meal, you must prepare yourself first. Your intention will be the difference between preparing food that will nourish you and others—or that will leave you feeling out of balance. Food is sacred. It's important to feel the great honor of preparing food and eating it. Saying a blessing or a mantra can help you feel more connected to the process. One of my young moms works in a sandwich shop and silently says a prayer over every sandwich she makes for each customer. If you do not feel up to preparing a meal, then don't do it. Prepare snacks ahead of time so that there is always a little something to eat in case you're not in the right frame of mind for cooking.

Sensual Food Preparation: When I talk about *sensual* food preparation, I'm talking about using all your senses in food preparation. Cuisine is the only art form in which you experience the artwork on all sensory levels in the process of creating it. Be mindful of each step and how you are engaging your senses.

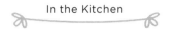

Let's practice engaging the senses while cooking.

- **Hearing:** Listen to the sounds in the kitchen, and select a playlist of songs that make you feel connected to this particular task.

- **Smelling:** Note the scent and choose aromatic spices to bring out more scent and flavor.

- **Tasting**: Don't be afraid to munch on the food throughout the meal prep process.

- **Touching**: Be mindful of textures as you prepare your meal—are there crunchy and smooth elements, for example? Think about how the food will feel as you eat it.

- **Seeing:** Fully observe the ingredients, making a beautiful plated presentation.

Therapeutic Versus Comfort Foods: Therapeutic foods are ones that heal—that assist in the process of regenerating healthy cells, recharging the body, and general renewal. Comfort foods are those that meet an emotional need. For instance, if you experience a bad breakup, you crave sweets—perhaps due to the lack of sweetness on a primal level in your life. Therapeutic foods like greens, nuts, avocado, and blueberries will balance out the system whereas traditional comfort foods that are starchier or sweet/salty will send you into big craving territory.

Useful Preparation Methods

Preparing our food doesn't just mean cooking. There are many ways to render food while maintaining its nutrient balance. Every now and again I get a vegan client who is interested in going the full monty: completely raw. Right away I teach the following methods so that she is best equipped to prepare health-supportive

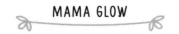

meals and snacks. Even if you are eating a lot of cooked vegan food, these techniques are great to have in your arsenal. I choose a diet that is 50/50 in winter (50 percent raw and 50 percent cooked), and 80/20 in spring and summer (80 percent raw and 20 percent cooked). I need the cooked foods to ground me and the raw foods to lift me up and spark my glow.

Dehydrating: Dehydration is a process by which low heat is used to dry foods. If kept below 108 degrees, that food is still considered raw. All of its nutrients and enzymes are still intact. This is a great way of getting bulkier foods into the diet that are nutrient dense, for example, dried fruits and flax crackers.

Fermenting: Fermenting is an anaerobic process (meaning a process that doesn't use oxygen) by which a food is preserved. Microorganism load increases when the sugars in the food are metabolized. If done on a small and less controlled scale, that is, spontaneous fermentation, the benefits are great. Large-scale production of pickles, on the other hand, results in a high acid content without a necessary increase in nutrition. Examples of fermented foods include kombucha, kefir, small-batch pickles, kimchi, and nut cheeses.

Soaking: Most of us have never learned this, but raw nuts and seeds—particularly ones with skin, such as almonds—should be soaked prior to ingesting. The soaking of raw nuts and seeds allows the enzyme inhibitors to release, rendering the nut or seed more digestible. To prevent a mean case of gas and to have the benefits of sprouted nuts or seeds, I suggest adding soaking to your program.

> **Glow Tip:** Soak nuts with skins for a minimum of three, and up to eight, hours to release enzymes. Water should cover the nuts plus extend an inch beyond to account for expansion. Then rinse and spread across a tray lined with cloth or paper towels to air dry for at least three hours.

Sprouting: Sprouting a seed, nut, or grain will, in effect, cause it to grow. When you eat sprouts, you are eating the vital potential of a new plant. There is a lot of life force in the budding sprout that gets transferred to your own body—and the life sprouting in your belly! Some yummy sprouts include sprouted quinoa, mung beans, lentils, and chickpeas. Sprinkle sprouts over salads or add half a cup to your smoothie to pump

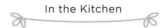

up the volume on protein. If you're running short on time you can purchase sprouts at your supermarket, Asian market, health-food store, or local green market.

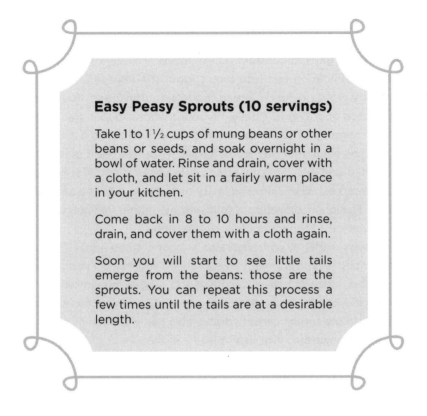

Easy Peasy Sprouts (10 servings)

Take 1 to 1 ½ cups of mung beans or other beans or seeds, and soak overnight in a bowl of water. Rinse and drain, cover with a cloth, and let sit in a fairly warm place in your kitchen.

Come back in 8 to 10 hours and rinse, drain, and cover them with a cloth again.

Soon you will start to see little tails emerge from the beans: those are the sprouts. You can repeat this process a few times until the tails are at a desirable length.

Going Dough-*Nuts*!!

Anyone who knows me well knows about my love affair with bread. I don't make a habit of eating it daily, and I don't keep it in the house. But get me in an Italian restaurant and pass me the basket of hot bread and olive oil and it's OVER! I've loved bread for as long as I can remember. When I was pregnant with my son, I indulged in the various gluten-free varieties. My favorite is millet bread.

I know—sounds contradictory, right? I've talked in earlier chapters about cutting out white flour, which is of course the main ingredient in bread. And I do believe in going gluten free as much as possible. But that doesn't mean I don't appreciate how good bread is! I just eat mostly gluten free and in moderation.

Flour products contain a mix of substances—processed grain, fats, and sugar—that trigger cravings. Pastries, cookies, and bread cause rapid elevation in glucose and insulin, which we have already discussed can result in gestational diabetes. Flour products also tend to be loaded with calories, contributing to weight gain. Many of them contain a fair amount of salt, which dehydrates your cells and causes blood vessels and organs to contract. These foods provide a short-term feeling of relaxation and gratification because they trigger the release of serotonin, which makes you feel warm and fuzzy. Bread, bagels, muffins, and flour products are the leading source of cravings. Really, I wonder whose idea it was to serve toast with jam in the mornings. The combination of sugar and carbs is a recipe for a shit show. Just imagine what your day would be like if you started it off with a big pack of Skittles. Well, bread and jam or pastries is the equivalent: it spikes your blood sugar and delivers a sense of calm and levity primarily due to the serotonin release from the brain. This quick elevation is followed by a rapid decline, which results in low energy, anxiety, and for some of us, depression.

The good news is that all carbohydrates are not created equal. The blood sugar response I described is typical when you eat refined sugars. As I've said before, complex carbohydrates, which include whole grains and veggies, burn more evenly through your system. So they don't precipitate spikes and plunges in your blood sugar.

Processed (simple sugar) carbohydrates also carry a much higher calorie load than complex carbohydrates. For example:

Slice of Bread: 1,120 cal/lb
Broccoli: 130 cal/lb

Hello, that's huge! You can literally graze as much as you want on green glow foods like broccoli and still not surpass the calories you'll find in a slice of bread. Just something to keep in mind when making food choices. If you are longing for starchy satisfaction try adding half a cup of brown rice or a slice of gluten-free bread to your meal.

Another reason to avoid bread and other flour products is that they contain wheat. About 30 percent of my clients are gluten intolerant or suffer from celiac disease, a disease that makes the small intestine hypersensitive to gluten. I find that when I don't eat wheat products I feel great. But when I indulge in a piece of bread I feel a set of familiar symptoms that remind me why I rarely eat it in the first place. For some, these symptoms are subtle and may include bloating, indigestion, constipation, headaches, fatigue, insomnia, depression, and—last but

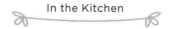

not least—excessive mucus. For others the symptoms are more amplified. But the truth is, wheat is not great for any of us. If you're not convinced on the gluten front, consider this: wheat is high in phytic acid, which interferes with the absorption of minerals, especially zinc. After all the effort you're going through to nourish your body and your baby, why mess with things by eating wheat?

Kiss My Atkins

The Atkins diet and others like it are high in protein and fat, and low in carbo-hydrates. These types of diets were originally prescribed for weight loss. I had a high-performance athlete client who was on a full-blown Atkins regimen when we started working together. She was early into her pregnancy and wanted my servic-es in meal planning and preparation to make her first few months move smoothly. As a vegan, I believe in peppering the lives of others with amazing plant-based cuisine, which is what I did to balance her diet out.

High protein consumption can damage the kidneys and contribute to blood loss and osteoporosis—which is so unsexy. What's more, high-protein diets tend to be high in cholesterol as well, which contributes to heart disease. In spite of the fact that they are linked to weight loss, it's my take that such diets are harmful (and at the very least, constipating). I want you to steer clear of this diet—especially during pregnancy and postpartum. Let me break it down for you, sister.

When you consume excessive protein from animal products, you fool your body into thinking it's starving by depriving it of carbs—the body's fuel of choice. In response, the body shifts into ketosis—abnormal fat metabolism mode. Ketosis is an emergency situation, where the body is forced to convert fat into ketones. Once detected, the body will burn protein for a few days. Protein is the primary constituent of muscle, so it's not a good idea to burn it. High-protein diets also reduce hunger so you tend to eat less, keeping the blood sugar and insulin levels low so you keep burning fat. It sounds like a bonus—except you are not looking to burn fat right now, you're pregnant!

Rather than an all-protein diet, I suggest *downsizing* your protein intake. I say this because once consumed, protein converts to acid in the body. The more ani-mal protein you eat, the more acidic you become. When that acid pours into the bloodstream, the body has to work overtime to alkalize the blood pH by releasing its own natural alkalizing agent: the phosphorus from your bones. When the phos-phorus goes out the door, your calcium leaves with it. Bones become weaker and more porous, leading to osteoporosis—which is not the result of a milk deficiency, as so many of us have been taught, but is the result of excessive protein consumption in the diet leading to a highly acidic bloodstream. Excess animal protein also converts to ammonia, a ragingly toxic chemical. Low levels of fiber mean that hormones are elevating, which we don't want. Fiber binds with hormones like estrogen to carry the excess out of our system.

Americans eat six times the amount of protein our bodies need for proper metabolic functioning. A more moderate 3 to 4 ounces of protein a day delivers enough tyrosine to the brain to stimulate production of the dopamine and norepinephrine we need to keep us mentally acute. Protein is used by the body for cell replacement and repair. Quiet as it's kept, you can get all the protein you need from a vegetarian diet. Doctors won't share that information with you and often will wonder how you get your protein. Plant foods contain all the amino acids needed to produce complete proteins. The World Health Organization says that pregnant women need only get 6 percent of their calories from protein, and lactating women should get 7 percent of their calories from protein. Children need no more than 5 percent of their calories from protein. A glow foods diet provides more than 7 percent without any animal products. So now that you know protein doesn't have to come from animal products, you can show off at your next prenatal visit. When your practitioner asks how you're getting your protein, you can just say "from my vegetables, of course!"

Mindful Eating Practices

I grew up in a household where we sat at the dinner table for meals, drinking while eating was forbidden, and most of our food was fresh. We were not allowed to watch television or talk on the phone while eating and even now I uphold that mindfulness ritual in my own home. My maternal grandmother taught me the value of prayer, and I developed a regular practice of blessing my food. When I first started eating mindfully as a teenager I was really interested in slowing down and chewing more so I could notice when I was full. It's all about connecting with your environment, the people, and the food—and that excludes your iPhone or your BlackBerry.

My starting suggestion is to take five to ten long deep slow breaths before eating a meal. Just this modest shift reduces stress and turns on your full digestive power. It's like hitting the RESET button for your nervous system. When we are stressed, we don't digest. Our food ferments in our bellies. (And not the good kind of fermentation I mentioned before!) Breathing is a way for us to slow down and be present. The next step is to literally become a slow eater. The more you chew, the more the palatine glands (located in the back of the mouth, on either side of the tongue and closely associated with the palate) are stimulated. Those masses of lymphatic tissue known as the tonsils lie beneath the lining of the mouth and, like other lymphatic tissues, they help to protect the body against infections. The 32 teeth chewing and clattering activate your 33 vertebrae and energize the nerves. This act of chewing sends signals to the brain about our hunger. The brain can tell us much more effectively that we are satisfied when we eat slowly and breathe deeply.

I remember watching how my mom would linger over her meals: eating slowly, laughing, engaging in meaningful conversation, and stopping once she was full. In our family she was the target of many jokes because of her tortoise-style eating habits. Yet she instilled in us slow eating patterns that I share with my own son today.

Many digestive issues, including reflux, could be alleviated by simply slowing down and chewing our food more carefully. Also, take the time to observe what happens in your body after eating. Notice if you experience gassiness, fatigue, fogginess, or if, on the other hand, you feel energized, calm, and satiated. Your food is loaded with information and will reveal to you whether or not you should be eating it; it's up to you to listen. The enteric nervous system of the gut holds a huge amount of intelligence. When you eat too swiftly, you miss your own gut wisdom. Take time to breathe through each meal and listen to your belly wisdom. Your body will in no uncertain terms indicate to you what is going on within.

Practice *dining*, not simply feeding, honey! Set the dinner table and light a candle—you deserve it. Sit in communion with family and friends, or savor a delicious meal by yourself. I dine every night with my son, Fulano, and I make sure to have breakfast with him, too. Those are two meals we never miss eating together. He says a blessing over our food that he came up with when he was three years old:

> Thank you for the food, thank you for fixing it, thank you for growing it, and thank you for picking it. Amen.

He is a great eater; he loves lentils, brown rice, seaweed, and avocado, and is a big fan of Asian-style cuisine because of all the condiments. He loves a good couscous tower with hummus, and soups and smoothies are his joy. His authentic relationship with food is a direct result of my food habits; he's following after modeled behavior.

Your baby is also learning about your diet in utero, as the amniotic fluid takes on the flavors of foods you eat. Believe it or not, by slowing down and being intentional about preparation and eating, you set the stage for your little one's eating habits. The next chapter will introduce a new prenatal yoga sequence leaving you swaying in the breeze.

CHAPTER 11

ON THE MAT

Glowing with the Flow!

I find that when women enter their second trimester, they are in a state of flow. They find their rhythm and things are more fluid. They feel less uptight and freer in their bodies. The first-trimester discomforts have passed, and there is now an influx of energy. These moms tend to feel a sense of strength and readiness for activity. I had a mommy-to-be who went from morning sickness to energy enthusiast seemingly overnight. She wanted an exercise that would keep her body supple but also tucker her out by evening time. I practiced yoga with her three times per week and signed her up for lap swim class for two days per week. It was exactly what she needed to balance the increase in energy and help her to tune inward.

This desire to move may come in reaction to the slower moving, less active first trimester. That's why I give second-trimester clients postures that address stagnation and the compression of our middle organs due to the increasing size of our bellies. Mama Glow flow yoga in the second trimester is meant to support movement of the body, blood, bowels, and lymphatic system. It includes squats, pelvic rolls, and spinal flexion, also known as Cat/Cows.

Here is the Mama Glow sequence for second trimester, which you can practice daily. It will only take you 15 minutes, depending on how long you stay in each posture. You will need a yoga mat and a set of blocks. You can find this sequence in a video at www.mamaglow.com.

Mama Glow Second Trimester Yoga Sequence

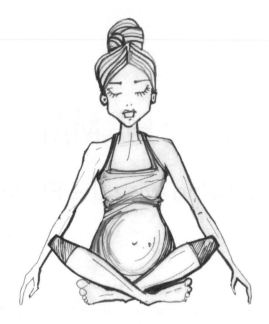

Grounding Sequence: This warm-up sequence helps strengthen your arms, increase respiration, loosen and increase blood flow to the hips, increase spinal mobility, and promote relaxation.

How to do it: Start seated with crossed legs, one hand resting on the belly and one on the heart. Close your eyes and tune inward. Notice what feelings arise. In your mind, watch the waves of the sea crash upon the shore. Find stillness within as you breathe.

Move into Pelvic Rolls: Place hands on knees and begin rolling your pelvis in circles, starting to make space in the pelvic bowl and inviting your hips to spread as you approach your final trimester. Switch direction.

Come to center again for Seated Goddess Posture: Sitting up tall, take the arms up on the inhale. On the exhale, take the arms open and down to the floor. Once again breathe the arms up, but this time bend to either side slowly and gently, strengthening the obliques and serratus anterior muscles in your sides.

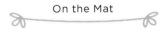

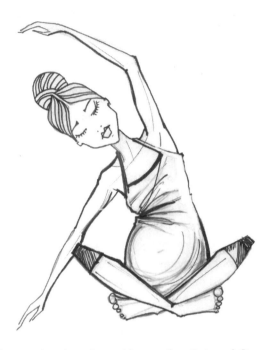

Next, roll forward to hands and knees for Cat and Cow: Move to your hands and knees in a table-top position. Align your shoulders, elbows, and wrists in one line, spreading the palm of each hand wide onto your mat with hands shoulder-distance apart. Keep the neck as a natural extension of the spine, and bring your gaze to the floor. On an inhale, curl your toes under, lifting your tailbone and chest toward the ceiling while dropping your belly toward the floor. Your gaze will be upward, toward the ceiling. Let the scooping movement in the spine initiate from the tailbone. On the exhale, release the tops of the feet to the floor, rounding through the spine and sending the belly toward the ceiling, stretching through the tops of the shoulders and dropping the head, so you are gazing at your navel. Repeat for 5 to 10 breaths.

Glow Tip: *Keep your arms firm and protect your neck by drawing your shoulders down your back and away from your ears. It's a rock-a-bye motion that gently rocks your baby inside your body.*

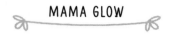
From hands and knees, push back to Downward-Facing Dog—the inverted V position. Shift the weight into your heels, relax your neck and drop your head. Pedal out through your feet as if climbing on a Stair-Master. As you inhale slowly, bend your knees and walk your hands backward toward your feet. When you can't go any further, slowly rise up to stand, vertebra by vertebra, allowing your head to come up last. Roll your shoulders back until you are standing straight and tall.

Standing Poses

Strengthen the leg and butt muscles that attach to the knees and pelvis. These joints are vulnerable during pregnancy because of the softening effect of the ligaments caused by the hormone relaxing. Strong supporting muscles will help protect the joints and prevent injury. Most important, standing poses help generate heat, physical fortitude, and confidence.

Standing Cat-Cow Series: This sequence encourages spinal articulation and strength in the muscles along your back and thighs, both of which will help support your growing body.

How to do it: Stand with feet hip-distance apart on your mat and have two blocks handy in case you need them. Start by standing upright, with feet parallel, in Mountain Pose. (For an optional boost, you can place one block between the feet to make sure that they remain parallel, and take the other block and place it between your thighs and squeeze throughout the posture. The action of squeezing the block width-wise between the thighs helps to tone the inner thigh muscles and bring awareness to the muscles of the pelvic floor.) Take a deep inhale and raise your arms perpendicular to the floor, palms facing each other, and as you exhale bend your knees parallel with the floor and send your hips back like you are sitting into a chair. This is called Awkward Chair Pose. To avoid overswaying the lower back, tuck the tailbone slightly toward the floor. As you bend your knees, take the thighs more parallel to the floor and feel your torso leaning slightly forward above your thighs. Arms continue to reach overhead, unless you have high blood pressure, in which case the hands can stay on your hips or parallel to the floor. Stay in the pose for 20 seconds, and then come out of it with an exhalation—rounding the spine with hands on your knees, relaxing your head toward your chest.

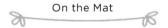

Resting your hands at mid-thigh with knees bent, relax your shoulders down your back. On the inhale, bend your knees to send your belly forward and reach your right arm up. On the exhale, round your spine and take that arm down, relax your neck, and gaze at your belly. On the next inhale, send your belly forward with knees still bent, and reach your left arm up. Repeat ten times.

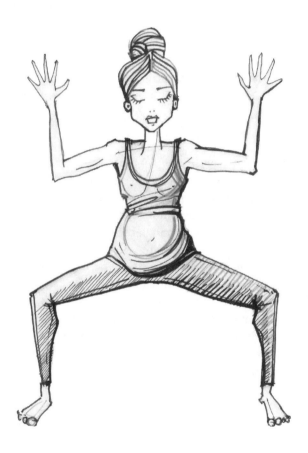

Goddess Squat Series: Strength in birthing squats is key. One thing folks fail to mention about labor is that you need to be in shape for it, especially your legs. This series gets your legs ready for the final stretch—the pushing phase. This squat sequence is the bomb for pregnant moms, because it helps to get our hips ready to deliver.

How to do it: Take the legs wide with knees slightly turned out. Inhale arms up overhead, and exhale, bending knees, bringing thighs parallel with the floor, opening arms out to either side, with palms facing up. Inhale up again, and repeat. Do this for about 20 counts.

Warrior II: This pose is particularly good for cultivating stamina and both mental and physical strength. It stretches the legs and ankles, groin, chest, ribs, and shoulders. It relieves low back pain and sciatica as well. It is important not to sway the lower back, which is common as the belly grows bigger and the uterus pushes forward. This pose is beneficial during pregnancy because it really gives a sense of warrior strength and confidence—strengthening the body, building a sense of endurance, and making sure that your mind can really focus. As you start to feel the sensation of the pose, remind yourself that you can get through anything as long as you move from breath to breath.

How to do it: Start with your feet parallel, hip-distance apart. Step your left foot back behind you at least one leg's distance. Then, turn your left foot out at a 60-degree angle with toes aiming forward, your right foot turned in slightly. Extend your arms to the side away from your body on a long inhale, bringing them parallel to the floor. Feel your chest open from your collarbone all the way up to your fingertips. As you exhale bend your front knee. Firming your thighs, bring the front knee directly over the front ankle, bringing that thigh parallel to the floor. The back leg is active, stretching from the inner thigh to the pinky side of your back foot. Allow your tailbone to drop and engage your back kneecap. Now, draw that thigh muscle up. Allow your breath to reach all the way down to your legs, down to your baby. Take a deep inhale and as you exhale straighten your front leg, keeping your arms extended (drop them by your side if you need a break). To do the pose on the alternate side: turn your front toes in and your back toes out, so you are reversing the position of the feet. Repeat with the left leg forward this time. To finish the pose, take a deep inhale and, as you exhale, straighten your front leg and step your back foot up to meet with the front leg, hands on your hips. Note: This is a great preparatory pose for Triangle, which comes next.

Triangle Pose: This pose strengthens the feet, ankles, and legs; elongates the spine, and arms; and opens the hips. It also allows the upper back to twist, releasing tension and stress. It stimulates the abdominal muscles as well. Many moms enjoy the inner thigh stretch and the feeling of lengthening chest, shoulders, and back muscles.

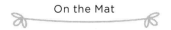
How to do it: Begin this pose from Warrior II. Straighten your front leg, toes pointing forward, and begin extending the torso by reaching the right arm forward, hinging at the hip crease, and rotating your torso up toward the ceiling. Reach the right hand down toward the floor, extending over the front leg. Draw the front thigh upward and tuck the hip as you come forward. Drop the right hand down onto your shin or ankle or a block, or if you are more flexible, onto the floor at the inside or outside of your right foot. The left shoulder stacks on top of the right as you open the chest, reaching the left fingertips up toward the ceiling, while keeping the left shoulder rooted in the socket. Gaze up toward the left fingertips. Then, draw the right thigh muscle upward, deepening the right hip crease. To come out of the pose: Rebend the front knee on the inhale and bring the torso back up to Warrior II. Reverse the feet, come into Warrior II facing the opposite direction, and repeat on the other side. When you are finished, go in to Downward-Facing Dog.

Dove Series: Here we will be stretching our hip flexors, outer hips, and groin muscles—as well as returning to the floor for a rest! The focus here is a posture many refer to as Pigeon Pose. As a New Yorker who is a little too well acquainted with pigeons, I prefer to call this one the Dove Pose!

How to do it: There is nothing more elegant than a mom-to-be in this posture. Start from Downward-Facing Dog. Step the right foot forward and place it just inside your left hand. Tip your knee to the right, until it touches the floor—just inside your right hand. (Your shinbone should be almost parallel with the front of your mat.) Keeping your hands in line with your knee, extend your chest forward, while supporting yourself on your fingertips. Try a few rounds of spinal flexion—waves of the spine—before resting your sitz bones, the bones you normally sit on, directly on the mat. You may also use a blanket or blocks underneath your hip to prop yourself up with a little support in this juicy pose. Once you are finished, return to Downward-Facing Dog and repeat on the other side.

With your pregnancy well under way, this practice will help to energize and revive your body from the inside out. For more fleshed-out sequences and a full video class to support the work you're doing in this book, visit www.mamaglow.com.

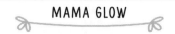

> Make a playlist of your sexiest music—music that makes you feel happy and free. Spend 20 minutes daily in solo dance, starting with moving your hips in circles. Circular movements help us to connect with the primal rhythms within. Close your eyes as you dance. Perhaps dance in dim light until you get more comfortable exploring flowing through dance. The movement awakens the body and inspires action in our lives.

Slow Birth

Slow birth is ecologically attuned, midwife- and doula-assisted care that respects the balance of nature. Over the past ten years the Slow Food movement has grown and gotten a lot of traction in the sustainable food community. Everyone speaks about slow food—how our food reflects the ecology of Mother Earth, how important it is to know where our nourishment comes from and how it's been cultivated, right down to the composition of the soil. Fresh, organic, local, seasonal food is our birthright. Since I'm in the birth business, I've thought a lot about this concept of *slow* as it can be applied to a new type of birthing model—one that is age old, but has gotten lost in the fast-paced world we live in.

Slow birth is not about the speed with which the baby emerges. Instead, it references the sum total of labor and maternal care practices we use. It means applying practices that are respectful that honor the inner ecology of the woman, her sacred anatomy, her innate wild wisdom, and her attuned rhythms.

Like slow food, slow birth is about getting back to the basics, celebrating what's natural. That doesn't mean birth without sophistication—in fact, it means listening to the sophisticated rhythms of the body. Sophistication doesn't always mean technological support! The body is highly sophisticated on its own, and it is capable of handling the whole host of processes required to bring forth a new baby.

The time of birth cannot be predicted. Such uncertainty can leave us and our medical practitioners uneasy. As a result, many women are encouraged to take medications like Pitocin to induce or augment labor, to "move things along"; but when our internal hormonal ecology is altered, we can become disconnected from what is happening in our bodies and even start to mistrust ourselves. No one

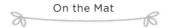

should govern the female body except the woman who lives in that body. When practitioners modulate the normal course of a labor (without a medical reason to do so), they perform an act against nature.

In my labor support work as a birth coach, or doula (Greek for "one who serves"), I strive to work with each of my clients to keep her in the flow of her hormones and in a rhythm with her baby. We use breathing techniques, visualization, sound, movement, essential oils, and therapeutic touch to help her labor comfortably. When you trust your body and have proper support, you can have an empowering birth. If slow food is a movement that takes us back to the land, with respect and honor for sustainable food, then slow birth takes us back to the womb—with respect and honor for the sacred birth process.

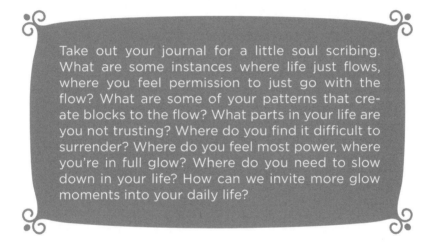

Take out your journal for a little soul scribing. What are some instances where life just flows, where you feel permission to just go with the flow? What are some of your patterns that create blocks to the flow? What parts in your life are you not trusting? Where do you find it difficult to surrender? Where do you feel most power, where you're in full glow? Where do you need to slow down in your life? How can we invite more glow moments into your daily life?

"Glowing with the flow" is really about allowing nature to take over. Let your inner-glow guru go crazy! When you let go, you soften. Get the mind out of the way and get into the body—the primordial self—so you can be face-to-face with your groovy goddess within. Stress keeps us from being in synchronicity with the universe. Being in touch with our internal spark, the divine glow of our inner goddess, will allow us to blossom.

CHAPTER 12

IN YOUR LIFE

Glow Potion Beauty Essentials

Beauty is an area that gets lots of attention during pregnancy—not always for the right reasons, however. Unfortunately, I come across women who are constantly on edge about their physical appearance during pregnancy. But during pregnancy we emanate so much beauty and sexiness. We're HOT! I briefly touched on beauty and self-love in Chapter 8, but here I want to address beauty and self-care practices that promote the glow. It's so important to take care of yourself and your skin while pregnant. And as Mama Glow Icon and natural-beauty maven Tata Harper, CEO of Tata Harper Skincare, says, a little pampering goes a long way. You read it right, if you do a little, your body will do the rest.

Those who know me know how much I love skin-care products. People always ask me what I use on my skin and how it looks so youthful. I'm about to let you all in on a little secret: I've been using Tata Harper Skincare products on my face for a little over a year now and I'm in *love*. I first came across Tata Harper's products through my gorgeous friend Denise Mari, owner of the raw food purveyor Organic Avenue. Talk about beautiful skin: Denise has been practicing raw veganism for years, before it was even popular. She's always on the cutting edge of what's hip and organic.

You may have heard of the so-called farm-to-fork movement. Well, Tata is leading the farm-to-face movement! Her products are chemical free and contain

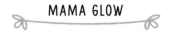
essences from plants that grow right on her lush farm in Vermont. The rest of her ingredients are wild-harvested in a few special places in the world where the land is well tended with organic and sustainable farming practices. With up to 29 active ingredients in each product, this line is no joke. Tata is a trained chemist from Colombia and a fierce mama of two. You can find her products online but together we've come up with some glow potions that you can make at home with glow foods right from your kitchen.

Skin Care

Skin care is something we take for granted. We want to look gorgeous, but often don't find the time to exfoliate and hydrate for the best quality skin. Get it together, honey. Take the time for yourself, your body deserves it!

My friend Jodie Becker Patterson of Georgia by G & Company, stresses the importance of cutting the harmful ingredients in your beauty products to optimize healing and maximize beauty for the entire family. As a mother of five, Jodie has never looked more amazing than she does when she is pregnant. In each of her pregnancies she was a walking billboard for beauty personified. Everyone can see that she pays close attention to what goes into her products. Product ingredients to embrace: plant extracts, essential oils, and herbs. Dirty ingredients to avoid include parabens, silicones, petroleum, mineral oil, artificial dyes, synthetic perfumes, and chemical preservatives. If you start to read the ingredient list and need to check the dictionary, then you should probably not be using it on your hair or skin. Much like we need to take charge of what we put into our bodies, we have to look at what we put *onto* our bodies. These lotions and potions we lather onto our skin penetrate; they don't just stay on the surface. Toxins that enter the bloodstream can pass through the placenta, so be mindful. Let your beauty shine through and use simple products or raw ingredients without the fuss. Check out the four recipes on the following pages for some healthy skin-care products.

Anointing Body Butter

1 cup shea butter
½ cup coconut oil
¼ cup sesame seed oil
    (raw, not toasted)
¼ cup evening primrose oil
¼ cup jojoba oil
10 drops of essential oil or fragrance oil

Put the shea butter and coconut oil into a double boiler. (Make your own double boiler by setting a glass measuring container on top of a canning ring in a saucepan, surrounded by boiling water.) Warm the butter and oil until soft but not melted. Remove from the heat and add the other three oils. Add the fragrance oil and then whip it up. I like to use my immersion blender for this task. Keep whipping until it is the consistency you want. Put into jars and cap. Voilà!

Sesame seed oil helps with inflammation and itching. Evening primrose oil helps in skin hydration. Apply the Anointing Body Butter to skin daily after shower to moisturize and protect your skin. This is especially helpful if you are living in a cold and arid climate.

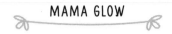

Tata Harper's Face/Body Scrub

Make a paste of equal parts honey, fine brown sugar, and oatmeal (half a cup of each one). Add 2 drops each of essential oil of grapefruit and essential oil of geranium. I work it all over my body, including my face. Scrub and rinse. This helps to deal with the dry and itchy skin and brings new skin to the surface in a gentle manner.

Skin Food = A Healthy Breakfast

Healthy breakfast at Tata Harper's house is a veggie plate. Sounds amazing! Chop enough veggies for four days. Harper likes asparagus, shiitake mushrooms, green beans, broccoli, and purple cabbage. Store them in a container in the refrigerator to make the morning routine easier and quicker. In a skillet, over very low heat, sauté 3 tablespoons of sesame seeds and sunflower seeds (slivered almonds work well, too). Next add in two handfuls of the chopped veggies and gently sauté until slightly softened, but still crunchy. Add a little bit of organic tamari.

This is how Tata keeps her glow, and she's taught me a lot of what I know about how to properly take care of my skin.

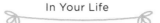

Latham's Coffee Sugar Scrub

$\frac{1}{4}$ cup ground coffee beans
$\frac{3}{4}$ cup brown sugar
1 $\frac{1}{3}$ cups olive oil or your virgin oil of choice
20 drops vanilla oil for fragrance

Mix all ingredients and spread over skin as a scrub. Rinse and pat skin dry.

After the scrub, I encourage a personal pampering practice of massaging the belly, hips, and breasts with the oil mixture above, or an emollient cream that has a base with something like shea butter or mango butter. You can also have someone special do this for you.

Hydrating Facial Masque

This hydrating mask feels so good you could eat it . . . you actually can eat it. Avocado based and yummy to boot, this mask will restore moisture to your skin. Don't forget your neck and upper chest. The French say the face ends at the breasts, so give your bust a little love, too, if you're in the mood.

Take an avocado and about ten drops of almond oil and whip with a spoon, then apply to face and neck. Let sit until it dries, then rinse with tepid water.

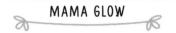

Natural products for face and body, and green alternatives for self-care are key. Thanks to sites like www.nomoredirtylooks.com, we can learn about the importance of quality chemical-free products. Spirit Beauty Lounge (www.spirit beautylounge.com) is a great site for finding chemical-free alternatives to makeup and skin care. Making your own glow kit, which includes natural products that are safe to use during pregnancy, is a great way to edit down your products to what's really essential: a good exfoliant, mask, moisturizer, and oil. The oil is the skin's nutrition. These are absolute musts.

Skin Elasticity and Stretch Marks

There's a great deal of anxiety around weight gain and stretch marks during pregnancy. The skin tends to stretch gradually, allowing the body a little time to adjust to the change in growth. However, the rapid weight gain that happens toward the third trimester results in subtle—if not intense—stretch marks in many women. There are ways you can minimize the likelihood of stretch marks and lessen damage to the skin. The results vary from person to person, and depend largely on your genetics, diet, and lifestyle. One thing to keep in mind is that these marks are the sign of a rite of passage that you've taken as a new mom. It's no sign of failure or inferiority; it's a sign of motherhood.

> **Glow Tip:** *Don't be fooled by the cocoa butter craze, studies show that it is not effective against stretch marks.*

Here are some ways to prevent stretch marks.

- Apply aromatic oil daily (see recipe on the next page).

- Exfoliate your skin often. Try basq's citrus sugar body polish or check out our recipe on the previous page and make exfoliation a part of your weekly beauty routine.

- Take vitamin E to increase skin elasticity.

- Apply vitamin E, shea, or mango butters to the belly, hips, and breasts in a circular motion. Be sure to massage the underside of

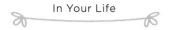
the belly as that is the skin that tends to overstretch the quickest. Vitamin E is very sticky and viscous, so mix it with your butters to create a powerful moisturizer that is smooth and absorbs well. This is best done in the evening after a shower, when your pores are still open.

- Get your proper intake of EFAs (essential fatty acids). These consist of flaxseed oil, borage oil, blackcurrant seed oil, sunflower seed oil, blue-green algae, and so on. Polyunsaturated fat is prone to oxidation, which leads to rancidity and free-radical generation, so store your fats in the refrigerator and consume them in balance with your other foods.

- Eat nuts and seeds (Brazil nuts, macadamias, almonds, walnuts, hempseeds, sunflower seeds, chia seeds, pumpkin seeds, flaxseeds). The oils from nuts and seeds help to nourish the skin from the inside, helping to increase skin elasticity.

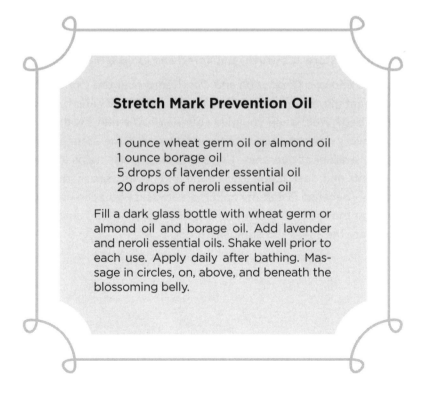

Stretch Mark Prevention Oil

1 ounce wheat germ oil or almond oil
1 ounce borage oil
5 drops of lavender essential oil
20 drops of neroli essential oil

Fill a dark glass bottle with wheat germ or almond oil and borage oil. Add lavender and neroli essential oils. Shake well prior to each use. Apply daily after bathing. Massage in circles, on, above, and beneath the blossoming belly.

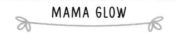

Hair Care

My favorite shampoo is made by a Brooklyn woman in her kitchen. It's an herb-al shampoo that is completely natural and safe for both my son and me. Better yet, I know and can pronounce every ingredient in it! It's called Royal Rinse by Herb N Life Productions, and you can purchase it online. Or you can whip up some glow potions of your own using these amazing tips for natural hair care. Following are a few of my favorite tricks.

- *Apply Sesame Oil to Reduce Sun Damage.* I'm a sun-baby but I know my beloved rays can be damaging to hair, causing it to become dry and brittle. Sesame oil provides excellent protection from UVA and UVB rays. Use raw, untoasted oil and rub into the hair and scalp before going out for long periods in the sun. You can even boost the oil with carrot seed essential oil, which is high in antioxidants.

- *Raw Apple Cider Vinegar Makes Silky Hair.* This is an astringent solution that tightens the hair cuticle. A tablespoon can be added to a deep conditioning treatment to tonify the hair, helping with silkiness and sheen. You can find raw apple cider vinegar in the health food store; it's usually unfiltered and looks a bit cloudy.

- *Brush to Improve Circulation and Oils.* Remember the stories of your great grandmother brushing her hair 100 times and braiding it before bed? Well, when you give your hair 100 strokes with a bristle brush every day, you stimulate the circulation in the scalp and give the hair a silkier appearance. Regular brushing also helps to remove pollutants and dust. If you are like me and haven't brushed your hair in years—because I wear my hair in dreadlocks—you can use oils to massage the scalp. You can also use eucalyptus-based shampoo to invigorate the scalp and stimulate blood flow.

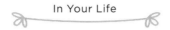

Making Your Own Glow Kit for Beauty Care

I believe in finding products you love and mixing and matching with some homespun goodies that help you to feel well pampered. Mama Glow must-haves for beauty:

- ☐ Facial Scrub
- ☐ Body Polish (sugar-based as mentioned earlier)
- ☐ Hydrating Mask
- ☐ Rose Water Mist
- ☐ Herbal Bath Soak
- ☐ Cream or Oil for Moisturizer
- ☐ Hair Wash
- ☐ Lip Balm
- ☐ Aromatherapy Oil

I keep all of these handy in my medicine cabinet in the bathroom—and even keep some of them in my purse! Rose water mist, lip balm, and aromatherapy oil all travel well. For more Mama Glow skin-care recipes visit www.mamaglow.com.

Glow Tips for Beauty

Veronica Webb, supermodel, TV personality, entrepreneur, and mother, is a deeply spiritual woman and Mama Glow Icon who balances lifestyle effortlessly while maintaining a fabulous glow. Veronica has two glow tips for beauty during pregnancy and beyond.

- *Sweat It Out Every Day.* Your body pulls all the toxins from inside to the outside through your skin.

- *Lather.* Moisturizing your skin twice daily is also super important as it's your body's largest organ and you want to protect it. Every choice you make should add up to your health.

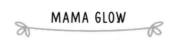

Beauty is generated from within. You must cultivate self-care practices that make you *feel* beautiful and you will project that outward. Put on a playlist and apply a face mask, I bet you will feel totally different 20 minutes later. In the next section you're moving into the Third Trimester, weeks 28–40. You are officially in the home stretch, baby, you will soon meet your little bundle of joy. It's glow time!

PART IV

IT'S GLOW TIME!
THIRD TRIMESTER
(WEEKS 29–40)

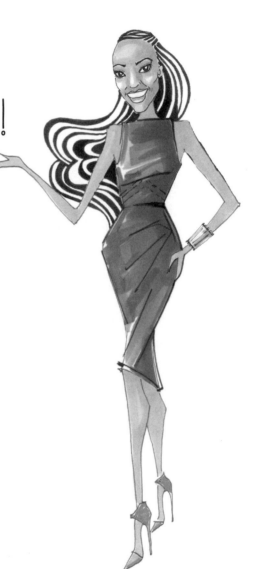

CHAPTER 13

THE HOME STRETCH

Glow Zone

You're almost there, mama! Just a couple weeks to go and you will meet your baby for the first time. Your body is getting ready and the baby is gaining weight. You may begin to experience "practice" contractions—called Braxton-Hicks contractions. When an expectant mom calls me with Braxton-Hicks contractions and she is preterm, I first try to rule out dehydration before assuming she is in early labor. If you feel signs of contractions and you're not in your late-third trimester, immediately start to drink water and contact your health-care provider.

You may also have an urge to clean your home, buy cute receiving blankets, and generally make way for baby. You will likely start to feel like you need to slow down a bit, to relax and enjoy these last few weeks before you give birth. Get some good rest, honey. Take it from me—they don't call it labor for nothing! In this chapter we explore the birth, the brain, and your labor. Common third-trimester discomforts like edema, itchy skin, and leg cramps will be addressed here as well. In this section you will get familiar with birth coaches, birth bags, and labor hormones. Baby's almost here—let's get started!

A Glance at Baby's Development in the Third Trimester

- *Week 31:* Baby is going through major brain development; her irises react to light and all five senses work now.

- *Week 34:* Baby recognizes and reacts to simple songs, and she will even remember them after birth. She pees about a pint every day—wow!

- *Week 36:* Baby is officially full-term and can be born as early as this week. Get ready!

- *Week 37:* Your full-term baby is gaining about an ounce daily and getting meconium ready for her first poop after birth.

- *Week 39:* Baby's brain is still developing rapidly. Any day she will be born, covered in vernix—a protective cottage cheese–like coating over her skin.

Mama's Development in the Third Trimester

The third trimester is a reflective period. You will soon be thrust into motherhood. Meanwhile your body is preparing for your labor—your hips spread and the baby drops deep into the bow of your pelvis. You may notice that moving more slowly through your day will feel better than trying to rush around. Emotionally, you are sensitive and should surround yourself with a tight sister circle—a network of women to support you postpartum—which I will show you how to create. You should also surround yourself with other loved ones who make you feel your best. It's a good idea to eat tinier meals at more regular intervals due to the compression of your middle organs. You may be totally turned off by sex, or this may be a time of total pleasure between you and your partner—each woman reacts differently, and either way, know that you are not alone. It may be important to you that your partner affirms your beauty and sexiness at this time, but it is more important for you to feel it from within. It's common to feel overwhelmed by your body's expansion. But like a friend of mine said, "Your belly and butt will never look this way again, embrace it!" I often recommend rubbing your belly in circles and saying the affirmation, "I love my fiercely beautiful body today."

Here in the home stretch you might notice that there is a lot of *stretching* happening in your body as well. Braxton-Hicks contractions are getting your uterus ready for showtime. I call it dress rehearsal. These contractions, named after the English doctor who first described them in 1872, can be mild or moderate, lasting for a few minutes or a few hours. They are essentially painless, but as you progress in your pregnancy, Braxton-Hicks contractions can mimic the sensation of early labor contractions, which makes it hard to distinguish them from preterm labor. Unless they are rhythmic, increasing in intensity, and growing closer together, chances are slim that you are in actual labor.

If the waves of Braxton-Hicks contractions are getting a little uncomfortable, try one of these simple measures:

- Take a warm bath. This will help the body relax.

- Change positions. You might find relief by positioning yourself differently.

- Drink a few glasses of water. As I've talked about throughout the book, dehydration can cause uterine contractions.

If you are not yet at weeks 36–37, keep an eye out for these signs of preterm labor. If you have any of these, it's time to check in with your doctor or midwife:

- If the sensations start to feel like abdominal pain or menstrual-like cramping

- If there is vaginal bleeding or spotting

- If there is an increase in vaginal discharge or mucus

- If you feel increased pelvic pressure, as if your baby is moving down

- If you have sharp lower back pain

If you are already at 36–37 weeks and you start to experience these symptoms, you can chill and relax until the contractions become more rhythmic before you call your doctor or midwife. In these last few weeks, it's expected that your body will be preparing physically for labor.

Top Four Third-Trimester Challenges

Itchy Skin and Rashes

These are common conditions, especially in the last three months of pregnancy, and they can be very uncomfortable. Itchy skin may be caused by an increase in estrogen. It usually disappears right after delivery. You may also find that things that normally make you particularly itchy—dry skin or eczema—can take you over the top with itching. To soothe dry skin:

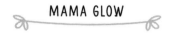

Anti-Itch Glow Foods: Brazil nuts, Hempseed oil, Pumpkin seeds

- Avoid using soap; it dries up natural body oils. If you don't want to eliminate soap altogether, try using an olive oil–based soap that will hydrate the skin as well as cleanse it.

- Use biodegradable natural laundry detergent or Chinese soap nuts. Generally speaking, they have fewer perfumes and gentler cleaning agents that prevent irritation of the skin.

- Wear cotton, hemp, and other natural fibers to keep skin cool.

- Apply strong moisturizers (shea butter, mango butter, cocoa butter, or coconut oil; see Chapter 12 for more information). Make your own at home, or try one of these sustainable and cruelty-free products: Mother's Blend by Mountain Ocean, Erbaviva Stretch Mark Cream, or coconut oil.

To Soothe Itching:

- Fill a muslin cloth or cheesecloth with one cup of oatmeal; tie it up and use it to wash yourself in the bath. You can add a teaspoon of each of these to the bath: lavender flowers, comfrey, and rose. For the best results, pulverize the oatmeal in a high-speed blender so it's like a powder, then make your sachet for the bath.

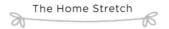
- Use chickweed cream or ointment.

- Use Bach Flower Remedies Rescue Remedy Cream.

- Take mildly steeped chamomile and Linden flower tea at night. I like the brand Hari Tea's Heart Center Calm.

- Load up on your EFAs to combat itchy skin: Take 2 tablespoons of flax or hempseed oil daily in a shake or salad dressing.

- Up your vitamin intake of zinc, selenium, and biotin, as well as B vitamins.

Edema

Whoa nelly, what's up with all the swelling? If you can't find your ankles and your feet are looking like loaves of bread, leaving flip-flops the only reasonable option for shoes, then you're experiencing edema. Edema results when the growing uterus puts pressure on your pelvic veins and your vena cava (the large vein on the right side of the body that carries blood from your lower limbs back to the heart). The pressure slows the return of blood from your legs, causing it to pool, which forces fluid from your veins into the tissues of your feet and ankles. Edema is most often an issue during the third trimester, particularly at the end of the day. It may be worse during the summer months especially where it's hot and humid!

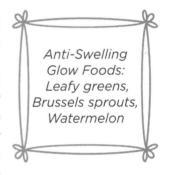

Anti-Swelling Glow Foods: Leafy greens, Brussels sprouts, Watermelon

What you can do to minimize swelling:

- Elevate your legs whenever possible. At the office it helps to keep a stool or pile of books under your desk.

- Relieve the increased pressure on your veins by lying on your left side, since the vena cava is on the right side of your body.

- Avoid crossing your legs or ankles while sitting.

- Stretch your legs frequently while sitting to get the blood moving: Stretch your leg out, heel first, and gently flex your foot to stretch your calf muscles. Rotate your ankles and wiggle your toes.

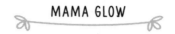

- Take regular breaks from sitting or standing. A short walk every so often will help keep your blood circulating.

- Wear comfortable shoes like Crocs or flip-flops that stretch to accommodate the swelling.

- Try waist-high maternity support stockings. Put them on before you get out of bed in the morning so blood doesn't have a chance to pool around your ankles.

- Drink plenty of water. The body retains water in the form of bloating when you are dehydrated.

- Avoid salty foods, fried foods, chocolate, white flour, sugar, and caffeine.

- Eat grapes, cucumbers, and watermelon to help deal with swelling. (See mouthwatering Watermelon Diva Salad recipe on page 173.)

- Exercise regularly, especially walking and yoga. Or try a water aerobics class—immersion in water may temporarily help reduce swelling, particularly if the water level is up near your shoulders.

Leg Cramps

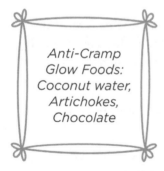

Anti-Cramp Glow Foods: Coconut water, Artichokes, Chocolate

You might have heard that leg cramps are a sign that you need calcium. My favorite supplement to recommend for leg cramps is a calcium-magnesium blend. That said, check with your health-care provider before taking any kind of supplement beyond your prenatal vitamin during pregnancy.

If you do get a cramp, immediately stretch your calf muscles. Straighten your leg, heel first, and gently flex your toes back toward your shins. It may be super uncomfortable at first, but it will ease the spasm and the pain will gradually dissipate.

You can also try to relax the cramp by massaging the muscle or warming it with a hot-water bottle. Getting up and walking around for a few minutes may help, too. Check in to make sure the cramps or pain is not a persistent tenderness in the leg. This may be the sign of a blood clot, which requires immediate medical attention. Blood clots are rare, but your risk is higher during pregnancy.

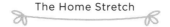
How to ease the cramps:

- Stretch your calf muscles regularly during the day and several times before you go to bed.

- Try prenatal massage and add heat to the region to help loosen the cramping tissue.

- Rotate your ankles and wiggle your toes when you sit, eat dinner, or watch television.

- Eat calcium-, magnesium-, and potassium-rich foods like bananas, blackstrap molasses, pecans, hazelnuts, and brown rice.

- Try a warm bath before bed to relax your muscles.

Varicose Veins

Varicose veins occur when your sluggish circulatory system is constricted due to the pressure of your growing uterus and the 50 percent increase in blood volume in the body necessary to support the growing fetus. This extra pressure makes it difficult for the teeny weeny valves in the vein to push blood back up to the heart. The blood pools and the vein puffs up and becomes more visible under the skin as a result. Exercises and yoga postures for your feet and legs may help improve circulation.

What you can do to improve leg circulation:

- Try massaging the legs and feet with warm oil, using long strokes upward toward the heart. This helps to move the blood from the pooled regions.

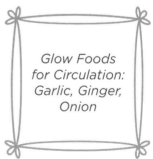

Glow Foods for Circulation: Garlic, Ginger, Onion

- Any form of cardiovascular exercise that uses the legs—for example, swimming, walking, and even dance—will improve the circulation.

- Take bromelain. This nutrient, which can be found in pineapple juice, aids in activating the breakdown of fibrin and helps to prevent blood clots.

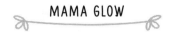

- Take 300–500 IUs of vitamin E every day to promote and improve circulation as well as ease pain. Please check with your doctor before supplementation.

- Take frequent rest periods when you're on your feet for long stretches.

- Avoid restrictive clothing and positions that might cut off your circulation.

- Sit in the cross-legged position whenever possible, and do daily pelvic rocking (moving in a circular and front-to-back motion using your waist and pelvis) exercises.

Nesting

Birds do it, and so do cats, apes, and other mammals preparing for birth. Nesting is an instinctual mechanism that prepares your "empty nest" to become full and quite busy for the next 18 years. Nesting is like spring-cleaning on steroids. Organization, cleanliness, and preparation are top priority. Not unlike how you cleared space to make this baby, now it's time to clear some more space for your soon-to-be bundle of joy. If you get hit with the nesting instinct as you're preparing for birth, make the most of it—now, before life becomes so hectic that even finding a moment to take a shower will be challenging.

Here's a bunch of last-minute details that you'll want to check off your list before going into labor.

Prep Your Essentials: For such little creatures, babies need so much. They go through more clothes, diapers, and creams than you can imagine. Stock up on baby soap, cotton pads, a rectal digital thermometer, rubbing alcohol, a nasal syringe, nail clippers, BPA-free bottles, nipples, and more. And for you, pick up plenty of super-absorbent maxi pads, witch hazel, Tucks medicated pads, and ice packs (not the kinds of things you want to run out of in the middle of the night).

Cook in Quantity: If your nesting instinct is accompanied by an obsession with cooking, take advantage and get your meal prep on. Make extra servings of your favorite freezer-friendly foods. Make soups, bake muffins, prep hot cereals and stews, and then store in single-meal containers in the freezer, clearly marked.

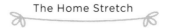

You'll be especially grateful to come home to homemade meals and snacks after spending time in the birth center or hospital!

Do Laundry: Wash your towels, duvet cover, pillow shams, throw rugs, guest sheets, and anything else that needs a once-over before the baby arrives. Use an alternative to hefty chemical detergents. I like Dapple products because they contain eco-friendly formulas that are safe for your family and the environment. If you live in a place where you don't have access to laundry, consider hiring a laundry service to take care of your needs for the first six weeks until you get into a rhythm. Stock up on your preferred detergent and cleaning solutions because you will be washing lots and lots of little onesies, pajamas, and receiving blankets.

Load Up Your Pantry: Stock up on staples like it's going out of style—because it is. You won't be doing the shopping once the baby arrives; you won't have time. It's all about keeping it healthy and convenient. Think nuts—the perfect nutrient-dense nibbler—trail mix, quinoa, and broths for easy soups. Other goods to get as you prepare for birth: whole-grain crackers, canned beans, brown rice, and healthy sauces.

Order Birth Announcements: You can get these online or at a stationery store, so they're ready to go as soon as you know the final baby stats. And address the envelopes now so they're ready to be stuffed and mailed.

Restock Your Refrigerator: Out with the old, in with the new! Throw away any outdated items and shop for fresh ones. Stock up on foods for breastfeeding that you'll want to have on hand once the baby has arrived—filtered water, fruits, veggies, hummus, prewashed salad greens, and so on. Make it easy on yourself and order your groceries online.

Spring into Clean Mode: You know the spring-cleaning that you're always putting off until next fall? Whatever the season, now's the time to tackle it while your nesting instinct is in full swing. Wipe down the windowsills and blinds, wash the floors, and vacuum under the couch and between the cushions—you may find a nice chunk of change while you're at it! Be sensible in your quest for cleanliness: call in a team of friends, blast some good dance music, and get moving. Use chemical-free cleaning solvents. I love the Mrs. Meyer's brand. Don't push yourself if you're pooped. Instead, push someone else, like your partner. Oh, and please stay away from ladders or other precarious perches! Stay as close to the floor as possible. In fact, hanging out on hands and knees scrubbing the floors Cinderella-style is not

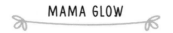
a bad idea. The position helps to open up your pelvis and the hip swaying encourages your baby to move down into the pelvic outlet.

Style Baby: Don't overbuy while you prepare for birth, but make sure you're well stocked on those newborn essentials (T-shirts, onesies, sweaters, and booties). Prewash baby's outfits so there are plenty of things for her to wear. If you haven't had a baby shower—put together a registry online to get all the basics and beyond.

Style Mama: Get fitted for the big day and postpartum. Buy nursing bras as well as nursing pads and easy-open (nursing) shirts. And stock up on soft, cotton, full-back underwear. Your thong days are over for a bit my friend. You'll need big bloomer action for the first few weeks after the birth. Don't go for the expensive undies here, as they may become stained with blood and discharge that will likely not wash away. Plan on tossing the granny panties about eight weeks postpartum.

Make a Who-to-Call List: Set up the list now, so your birth coach and partner know whom to inform of your new arrival. You can use it later to e-mail your birth announcement to your whole list. You can also set up a call chain, where you enlist five people who call five people who call another five people, and the information gets disseminated quickly and effectively.

Bedrooms, Birth Rooms: It's All the Same

The energy of the bedroom and birthing room is one and the same. What you do in the bedroom can help you in the birthing room. Yes, you read that right. (If you're totally confused just keep reading. I promise it will make sense in a minute.)

Have you ever noticed what it takes to get you in the mood for love? It may be dim lighting, slow music, the right scents, a clean and cozy space, a sexy voice, kissing, therapeutic touch, or erotic touch. The elements you use to get in the mood to open yourself up to an erotic experience—physically, emotionally, and spiritually—are the same elements that will make you feel comfortable enough to open up in labor.

Early on into my doula practice I came across a fierce diva who totally shifted my approach: Sheri Winston, the birth educator, sex educator, and pleasure vixen. She was teaching a workshop about ecstatic birth. I was intrigued, because I believed that my birth had been on the verge of an ecstatic experience. I canceled everything I had to do for the day to attend Sheri's workshop—and boy, did she blow my mind. One of the first things Sheri said to the group was "sex and labor

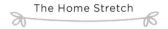

are the same thing." I looked around the room and everyone had a curious look on their faces. Sheri went on to explain how arousal and labor are almost the exact same physical state—from the neuropathways that light up to the hormones involved. In other words, orgasm and birth are the exact same state, structurally, neurologically, hormonally, and energetically.

Orgasm and pushing are related states. They are both primal experiences, part of what I call our "spiritual blueprint." They happen on their own, through the body's wisdom. That day at the workshop, Sheri went on to share with us how when you tilt your pelvis during intercourse there is a nerve response—a primal thrusting and friction. The uterus itself is a power player during arousal. It trains for labor by rocking back and forth during high-level arousal, promoting fertility and the opening of the sacred passageway. The round ligaments, which act as rubber bands keeping your uterus in place, are connected to the vulvic muscles of the vagina. They are also connected, via connective tissue, to your heart. When you climax, these body parts—vulva, uterus, and heart—are in total alignment. On its way out of your body your baby will hit the pudendal and pelvic nerves. (The term *pudendal* comes from the Latin word meaning shame—just another example of how culture has made sex dirty.) If you remain in a relaxed state as your baby descends, you may experience a combination of sensations that include tingling pleasure. Some women go even further, having a full-on orgasm at birth.

Sheri Winston says, "The more pleasure you allow yourself to experience prenatally, the more ecstatic a birth you will have." Access the sexual connection in early labor. This is when I encourage arousal between the couple. Encouraging the body to soften and open in the last few weeks of pregnancy will also prepare you big time for the big day. It's your last hurrah before the baby comes, so make time for intimacy! It may or may not result in sex. And sex is fine, as long as your membranes are still intact—that is, your mucus plug and amniotic waters are still in place.

In early labor, I encourage a lot of kissing. I had a birthing couple delivering twins who were so turned on in their labor that we ended up making a do-not-enter sign for the door so they could kiss and be comfortable while her labor quickly progressed.

As you learned earlier, the mouth and throat are hardwired to your pelvic floor and sacred passageway (birth canal). The opening of the mouth and throat signals the opening of the pelvic floor muscles and birth canal. So get ready to pucker up! Also, nipple stimulation will promote uterine contractions. So whether you are at home in the bedroom getting all steamy, or in the hospital birth room slow dancing with the lights dim, you can create the right circumstances to open up for your baby.

Brain Waves

Altered states of consciousness arise when you are in a dream, state of bliss, daydream, trance state, meditation, arousal, or labor. Western medicine thankfully can measure these altered states by measuring our brain waves. Brain waves allow us to understand our consciousness—giving value to an experience that is otherwise hard to measure. If you're driving a car with standard transmission you move between gears to alter your speed, right? Your brain-wave states function in a similar way.

Beta waves are the most common and highly valued by our culture. This is the brain-wave frequency you're tuned into while reading this book. This is the "thinking state," characterized by fast, erratic, short waves. You may be reading, but you are also thinking about your dry cleaning, what you want for dinner, and whether or not to go see that new romantic comedy. We are operating on beta waves during early arousal and also early labor.

Alpha waves are the state you enter into in meditation, daydreaming, or experiencing natural birth. Alpha waves are slower, more organized waves. They flow when we are doodling, and in a wakeful sleep state. This is the state that women need to be in to birth their babies. This state coincides with 0 to 4 centimeters dilation, in early labor.

Theta waves happen when there is no thinking—it's all about feeling. You drop right into the primal space and your ancestral wisdom kicks in. This is where many women experience what's called a "primal birth." This is also the brain wave you're riding when you cross the threshold of high-level arousal into climax (and multiple orgasm). When we get pulled into the vortex of our primal power, the labor takes over. The theta state coincides with mid-level to high-level arousal, or 5 to 6 centimeters dilation in active labor.

Delta waves are divine, literally. When your brain is functioning on this level you are experiencing cosmic bliss and oneness, or ecstatic birth. It may feel like an out-of-body experience. The waves of sensation are rolling through your body and you may have deep dreamless sleep and deep relaxation between contractions. You're experiencing whole-body feeling. This state coincides with the crossing of the threshold to transition, and full dilation.

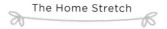

Pain is a reality and a necessary component of this process. That said, you can transform your pain into your purpose. The same way you relax into making love, you can relax into giving birth.

Giving birth is the ultimate rite of passage. Birth is an opportunity to explore your creative edge, your fears, and your courage. You come back from that experience changed. You should feel free to explore that power and give yourself license to go all the way in, to release the part of you that wants to control the experience and to trust the process instead.

Take a moment and gaze down to your belly. The miracle is unfolding every moment and although you are probably ready to meet your little one, remember that you will never have these moments again, so relish these last few weeks and snuggle up to your partner or close friends spending quality time before your baby arrives. In the next chapter you'll get a taste of comfort foods for your body and soul.

CHAPTER 14

IN THE KITCHEN

Comfort Foods

Brittany, a computer analyst, was pregnant with her first baby when she started to experience notable swelling in her hands and feet. It was a huge issue for her since she typed for a living. Suddenly she couldn't do her job! Immediately we lowered the salt intake in her diet and started incorporating foods that help ease swelling, including watermelon, cucumber, grapes, and pineapples. In this chapter we will explore powerful swell-quelling foods, anti-itch glow foods, and foods to ease cramping. These are what I call *true* comfort foods.

ARTICHOKES HEARTS, FAVA BEANS, AND SHITAKE SALAD
(4 servings)

With leg cramping more common in the final trimester, a great glow food to include in your diet is the artichoke. This heavenly recipe for warm artichoke salad will help. Artichoke hearts are rich in manganese, which soothes cramping legs and enhances thyroid function. Fava beans tonify the spleen-pancreas and kidney meridians, and flavorful shiitake mushrooms help lower blood cholesterol levels while boosting the immune system.

2 tablespoons olive oil

2 tablespoons ground cumin

1 teaspoon turmeric

1 bay leaf

8 ounces shiitake mushrooms, halved

1 pound fava beans, shelled

1 pound cooked artichoke hearts

2 tablespoons lemon juice

1 small bunch parsley, finely chopped

Sea salt and freshly ground black pepper, to taste

Heat olive oil over low heat in a large pan. Add the spices, then the mushrooms. Sauté for a few minutes, then add the fava beans with artichokes and ½ cup of water. Heat through and simmer until beans are tender, then add lemon juice and parsley. Season with salt and pepper and serve.

WATERMELON DIVA SALAD *(4 servings)*

This swell-quelling salad is the antidote to edema. If you are sensitive to onions, you can skip them and it will still be amazing. This seasonal salad is hydrating and cooling on warm summer days and helps to reduce swelling caused by heat, poor circulation, and edema. Watermelon is a powerful food, rich in vitamins A, B, C, lycopene, magnesium, and potassium.

One 5-pound watermelon

1 red or Vidalia onion

1/2 cup fresh chopped mint leaves

1/2 cup fresh chopped cilantro

1/2 cup fresh chopped parsley

4 tablespoons fresh lime juice

Salt and pepper, to taste

Cut the watermelon into 1-inch-sized chunks and place in a large bowl. Slice the onion into thin strips and soak in enough cold water to submerge the onions, for at least an hour. Discard the water and remove onions. Add the onions, mint, cilantro, parsley, and lime juice to the watermelon. Gently mix and season with salt and pepper.

GARLIC GINGER GREEN BEANS *(4 servings)*

Ginger and garlic are helpful ingredients in getting the blood moving and help-ing to improve leg circulation for varicose veins. This is helpful for people like me who always have cold hands and feet, too! Want to pack in some protein? Just add a cup of roasted almonds or tamari almonds roughly chopped to the dish. Now you're cookin', babe!

1 tablespoon olive oil

1-inch piece of ginger, peeled and grated or finely chopped

2 to 3 garlic cloves, peeled and crushed

3 cups green beans

1/2 cup nama shoyu soy sauce

2 tablespoons raw agave nectar or honey

2 tablespoons sesame oil

1/4 teaspoon crushed red pepper

1 cup almonds, chopped (optional)

In a large frying pan or wok, heat the olive oil and add the ginger and garlic, sautéing until lightly browned. Add the green beans, soy sauce, and agave nectar, and stir fry for 2 minutes. Remove from heat and stir in the sesame oil and the crushed red pepper. Top with almonds, if using.

Chocolate . . . A Love Supreme

A lot of moms punish themselves for wanting a snack, or for eating outside of the plan. Punishing ourselves takes up a lot of psychic energy. We are creatures of habit that don't like change. That's why the glow foods diet is not strictly regimented. It honors that our relationship with food changes over time. The glow plan is about paying attention to those cyclical changes, rather than setting food rules. Who we are has a lot to do with what goes on our plate. What are you bringing with you to the table—judgment, fear, intimacy, love? When you get over the need to be perfect, you can be present with the body. Developing body wisdom when it comes to food is all about listening to your body, which knows exactly what it needs, right now.

When you eat without mindful presence, you send a message to the brain that you are not satisfied. You'll only want more and more food. Our mood also has a powerful influence on how we process food. When we're stressed, the body can't digest food. The stress is a calcium depleter. It also lowers sex-hormone production. Cortisol, the most abundant stress hormone, desensitizes the body to pleasure. Pleasure is what you want to be experiencing most here in the third trimester, as you get closer to your blissful birth.

When we are looking to feel love, or get a "love reboot," the best nourishment is sometimes a piece of dark chocolate! The love affair we women have with chocolate is rooted in a biochemical connection. The most well-known love-related chemical is phenylethylamine, or PEA. It's a naturally occurring trace amine in the brain that acts as a neurotransmitter. PEA is a natural amphetamine. Just like the drug, it can cause stimulation. This natural upper contributes to that blissful feeling that comes with sexual attraction or your new baby. It gives you the energy to stay up all night talking to a new love or waking up to feed your little bundle every two hours. Sometimes this energy translates into the jitters; at other times, it simply keeps you wide-eyed, focused, and sharp, long past the time when you'd usually be in dreamland.

If you want to naturally help shift your mood—and treat yourself at the same time—have a square of dark chocolate. You don't need a whole bar, ladies! A small piece is enough to get the effect. It has to be the good stuff, though. Don't skimp and expect the same results from a Hershey bar. (Guess what? A Hershey bar has hardly any chocolate in it! Commercial milk chocolate bars contain more ilipe nut, cocoa extender, and emulsifiers than body products do.) Some of my fave chocolates include: Nibmor, Gnosis, Fine & Raw, Sweet Riot, and Green & Black's. Check out my chocolate shake on the next page, which is a nice treat and full of magnesium, which will get the bowels moving, too.

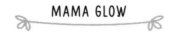

CHERRY BANANA SPLIT SMOOTHIE *(1 serving)*

This dessert smoothie has become a favorite. Frozen cherries, banana, and raw cacao nibs or cocoa powder can be used to create an otherworldly taste that takes you back to your childhood. The base is almond milk and you can of course substitute that for any milk variety of your choice. The potassium-rich banana and magnesium-rich cacao help prevent high blood pressure.

1 cup frozen cherries

1 ¾ cups almond milk (or milk of choice)

1 tablespoon cacao nibs or cocoa powder

½ banana, peeled

Place all the ingredients in high-speed blender and process until smooth.

I don't know about you, but all this comfort food makes me want to get cozy and relax. The next chapter takes you on a journey into restoration to ease the body, mind, and sprit in preparation for labor and delivery.

CHAPTER 15

ON THE MAT

Tune Out to Tune In

When mamas get to the final trimester I spend lots of time making them comfortable. Relaxing yoga postures to support this trimester include the Leg Drain, Reclined Cobbler's Pose, and Supported Bridge Pose. This trimester we're focusing on taking your practice off the mat and into the delivery room. You can bring your yoga practice into the birthing space and make good use of all the tools you have learned, all of which will help you explore ecstatic birth.

Some of the benefits of yoga during labor are:

- Yoga can help you connect with your breath. You can breathe in a way that is most natural and relaxing. This practice of moving your body rhythmically in tune with your breath while laboring is a powerful pain-management tool.

- Yoga can help move the labor along. When you practice yoga, you learn how to identify holding points in the body. If the body is tense, it will not move through the birth as easily as if it's relaxed. When our thoughts and body are tense, our breath becomes so; when we use yogic techniques to bring awareness to the body, relax our thoughts, and release our breath, the labor will flow.

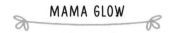
- Yoga teaches you about your body. Familiarity with how your body moves in different positions comes in handy when you're experimenting with positions during labor. You'll have an index of postures to move through to help keep you comfortable.

- Yoga helps you get to know your own voice. Vocalization is an important part of the laboring process. Most women move through labor using a variety of sounds: some high-pitched screeches and some deep-pitted moans. Sound in labor is a primal response to the overwhelming sensations that are happening within the body. Chanting in prenatal class allows an opportunity to become familiar with your inner Om.

Yoga is not just about asanas; it's about opening up and listening to your body. What feels good in the moment? What's needed? A *lok* is Sanskrit for a crystallized intention. We are holding the intention for a smooth birth and for life flowing within. It's visioning time!

If you have any props lying around, bring them onto the mat to help you get comfortable as you start visioning. Try a bolster or a birthing ball—a standard physiotherapy ball, for sitting or lying back in a reclined posture. Then focus on your visioning practice. What symbols or natural elements do you connect with? For some women, imagery of water—oceans, rain—helps them to *feel* more fluid. They embody that sensation of being weightless and boundless like water. You and your birth partner will want to practice visioning while still pregnant, as it is one of the most powerful tools for transforming and managing sensations of pain during labor.

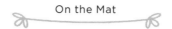

> To do this guided imagery for water, close your eyes and take five deep breaths—in through the nose and out through the nose. Get present in your body, and start to relax every part. Imagine yourself wading in warm waters in the sea. Notice the beautiful ocean floor. In the distance you see a wave forming. Watch it as it is coming closer. Notice any anxiety that comes up for you as the wave approaches. The wave is simply the surge of energy, a contraction moving through you that is helping to ease your baby down and out into the world. You begin to swim out toward the wave and as you paddle out with the current pulling you in, you get picked up into the vortex of the wave. You are riding the wave to shore. Once you arrive back at the shoreline, you rest for a few breaths, feeling the rush of energy and the strength of your body. Then you paddle back out to meet the rise of the next wave.

Make a list of images that you feel connected with and start writing your own guided visualizations that you want your birth partner to reference during your labor. Check out other guided meditations and audio on my website, www.mama glow.com.

Pump Up the Volume: Pelvic Pumping

Every woman should be doing these exercises and yet none of us thinks about it until we are about to have a baby. Very interesting! Our culture doesn't teach the art of the pelvic pump. Some people think I'm talking about Kegels, but it is so much more than that. *Vajroli Mudra,* or the "pelvic pump," generates intense energy in the lower body while keeping it contained. This builds up pressure in the energy channels. Once the containment is released, that pressurized energy shoots up the spine, breaking through any blocks or restrictions.

Vajra means thunderbolt in Sanskrit. Vajroli Mudra (the thunderbolt) stimulates the genitals with activated blood. Vajroli is simply the constriction of the

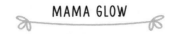

urethral, vulvic, and perineal muscles. Vajroli Mudra tightens vaginal walls, which will stretch considerably during childbirth, and allows great pleasure for both partners during intercourse. For most men this exercise is the solution to the problem of premature ejaculation. For women it is the means to a more pleasurable sexual experience. But this exercise also helps to get women familiar with recruiting the muscles required for pushing the baby out. And it is one of the first exercises you can do postpartum. Mastery of this exercise allows you to experience longer and more intense orgasm, and allows you to understand how to release your baby during your pushing phase.

The Elevator (Pelvic Pumps): Because pelvic pumps are so helpful, I always keep this exercise handy when working with pregnant moms. You're going to close your eyes and envision an elevator, wherever you like. (I like to pretend it's the elevator at Saks Fifth Avenue, or someplace fun like that.) Next you'll imagine the muscles of your vagina as that tall building. The base of your pelvic floor will be the bottom floor of the building, and your belly button is the top floor. You will slowly concentrate on raising the elevator by tightening your muscles from the "bottom floor" to the "top floor." At the top, you'll give a slight hold before bringing the elevator back down, slowly relaxing your muscles from top to bottom, counting the entire journey as one repetition.

How to do it: To start, sit up nice and tall on a chair or the floor. You can sit in Cobbler's Pose or with yoga blocks between your knees. Taking a few cleansing breaths, inhale and squeeze that elevator up to the first, second, third, then fourth floor. Hold all the muscles in as you draw up. Remember to breathe and check to be sure you aren't clenching your jaw. Then, slowly release the elevator down for 3, 2, 1 counts. Finally, go deep within and push out of the basement (where all the sales are)! Repeat for ten repetitions.

I can't tell you how many births I've attended where I've said push out through the basement and something clicks for moms and they remember how to push. Practice this daily, mama!

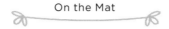

Relax and Restore

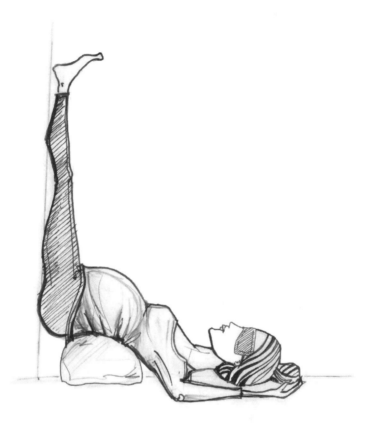

Leg Drain: This is the great mother of all restorative yoga postures. It combines the benefits of Corpse Pose with the gifts of a gentle inversion. This posture promotes rest. It will help drain any blood or lymph that has pooled in your legs, ankles, and feet, and gently lengthen the hamstrings. The floor provides a valuable feedback loop, allowing the spine to lengthen and stretch with maximum support. The sacrum is flattened to complete a graceful full-spinal extension, while the lungs are freed to empty and fill with ease—which is especially important when you are getting further along in pregnancy. Folded blankets may be used beneath the sacrum or under the length of the spine to provide support and enhance a deeper union with the breath.

How to do it: Bring your hips within a foot of the wall and lie on your left side. Send your right leg up the wall and, rolling onto your back, slide the left leg up to meet the right. Your hips can be slightly away from the wall, creating a 45-degree angle with the legs. Close your eyes and relax your shoulders, then breathe deeply. Stay here for a minimum of five minutes.

Glow Tip: If you hang out here for 20 minutes, it's equivalent to taking a two-hour nap! You are welcome to practice this pose up until 36 weeks, after that point it is advised not to enter this pose because of the pressure that might be placed on the vena cava.

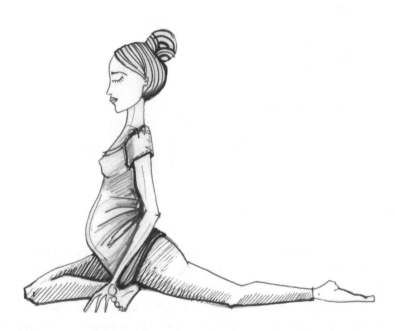

Pigeon (or Dove Pose): This pose—which we also used in the second trimester—is great for those who have any low back pain, tight hips, or sciatica. It helps lengthen the hip flexors and stretches the groin, thighs, chest, shoulders, and neck, and it stimulates abdominal organs.

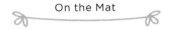

How to do it: Start in Downward-Facing Dog. As you inhale, bend your right knee up, sliding the leg forward all the way to the front of your mat. Let the outside of the right shin rest on the mat. Slowly slide your left leg back, straightening the knee and descending the front of the thigh to the floor. Position the right heel just in front of the left hip. Then slide your hands back toward the right shin and push your fingertips firmly into the floor. Lift your torso away from the thigh. Open your chest. Stay here for a couple of breaths. Then slowly bow your torso forward, walk your hands out in front of you, and come to rest the forearms on the floor (your belly may touch the floor here). Stay where you feel comfortable and take 10 deep breaths. Coming out of it, plant the hands and step the right leg back to Downward-Facing Dog. Repeat on the other side.

Reclined Cobbler's Pose: This wonderful pose allows you to relax the entire back, provides a supported stretch in the hips, and opens the chest to create more space for deep breathing. Enter a total state of calm here. This posture can be practiced throughout your pregnancy.

How to do it: Using a support bolster or blankets, create a stack that's about one foot off the ground. Sit in front of your support with your sacrum touching the base. With your knees bent, press your feet into the floor. Place your hands to the floor outside of your hips. Gently lie back over the support of your bolster or blankets. You should feel a release in the lumbar region of the spine. Then slowly slide your knees out to either side and bring the soles of your feet together to touch. Close your eyes and rest here, taking full, deep breaths. Coming out of the pose, bring your knees together and slide them over to the left side. Take your hands to the floor and push up to sit.

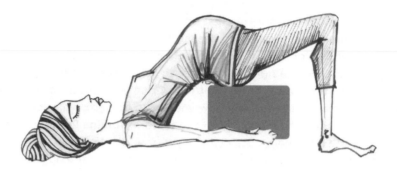

Supported Bridge Pose: The anatomical focus of this pose is the uterus. The Supported Bridge stretches the chest, neck, and spine and allows you a gentle back-bend with total support. Some of the benefits include stimulation of the abdominal organs, lungs, and thyroid; improved digestion; and reduced anxiety, fatigue, backache, headache, and insomnia. This pose calms the mind and helps alleviate stress and mild depression. This is a great pose for postpartum moms as well.

How to do it: Lie on your back, bending the knees and pressing the soles of the feet into the floor. Bring the feet parallel and hip distance apart. Have a yoga block on hand. Lift your hips and slide the yoga block directly under your sacrum. Rest your sacrum on the block and allow your arms to rest alongside your body. You may stay here for a few minutes. To come down, lift the hips and slide the block out from underneath you. Lie on your back and draw your knees in toward your chest, then roll over to your left side and rest.

Making the time to relax and find comfort in these last few weeks is key to maintaining well-being. You don't need much, just a quiet space and a willingness to relax and open up—this will be helpful when you are in labor. Now that you have the insightful tools for relaxation, let's take the birth journey. In Chapter 16 you'll learn everything you need to know for your blissful birth!

IN YOUR LIFE

Your Blissful Birth

As we talked about in Part III, getting educated on birthing alternatives—from home birth to hospitals—is one primary focus of the second trimester. Now that you've chosen your birth team, it's time to really drill down into your birth plan.

What is a birth plan? It is a simple, clear outline of your preferences for labor and delivery. Beyond being a useful visioning tool, a birth plan helps everyone on your team understand your wishes. Everyone who will be supporting you can read it and get on the same page when it comes to your labor and newborn care. The birth plan covers everything from pain management options during labor to post-partum sleeping arrangements. It communicates your preferences and helps the rest of your birth team jump on board with your wishes.

I have included a birth plan in Appendix D that addresses the spectrum of options for home, birth center, and hospital births. Fill it out to help clarify your preferences for your labor. I'm actually not a big fan of calling it a plan, because birth is one of those things that is out of our control. Instead, think of it as a visioning exercise. It will help you get clear on what you would *like* the experience to be, and to explore and learn about all the possible outcomes. The result is that you will be prepared for whatever comes on the big day. You can fill out this five-page birth plan in Appendix D or go to my website for a digital version, www.mamaglow.com.

Some birth coaches' general service offerings might include the following:

- Prenatal Visit(s)

- Birth Preferences (sometimes called Birth Plan) Assistance

- Recommended Reading

- Lending Library of Books and Videos

- Telephone Support

- On-Call Support 24 Hours a Day

- Continuous Labor, Delivery, and Postpartum Support

- Initial Breastfeeding Assistance

- Postpartum Visits

- Backup Doula Support

- Referrals for additional assistance, as needed

Birth Coaches are the Bomb!

Call me biased, but I think every mama-to-be should explore the option of having a birth coach as part of her birth team. A labor support coach, or doula, is a woman who mothers the mother. She offers continuous support and constant presence for the laboring mother. After attending so many births, these coaches have deep wisdom, comfort, and encouragement to offer. Not only are birth coaches trained to provide the best in support, but they also help liaise between the doctors, nurses, and your partner during the process. She has a lot of experience keeping the family unit calm, while serving as an educator, advocate, and cheerleader for the laboring mother. She's the binding agent that helps keep it all together!

The doula can coach the laboring mom in breathing, relaxation, movement, and positioning. She also assists families in gathering information about the course of their labor. Labor support usually includes prenatal and postpartum meetings or home visits, 24-hour on-call support, massage and counterpressure during labor, help with positioning for the mother's comfort, and facilitation of fetal descent and rotation. Not to mention photos of your baby immediately after birth!

Birth coaches help facilitate an easier birth. In fact, having one present at your birth can cut your laboring time by 50 percent! Now if that's not incentive to look into getting a doula, I don't know what is. When I gave birth I didn't understand the value of having a birth coach present. I did however have four of the most wonderful staff present, as well as a midwife-in-training, since mine was the only birth at that time. According to *Mothering the Mother,* by Marshall Klaus, John Kennell, and Phyllis Klaus, studies have shown that the physiological effects of continual support during labor reduces the chances of needing a C-section by 51 percent, reduces length of

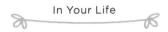
labor by 25 percent, reduces use of analgesia by 35 percent, reduces Pitocin augmentation by 40 percent, reduces the use of epidural anesthesia by 60 percent, and reduces use of forceps and vacuum by 30 percent.

Moms who work with doulas report greater satisfaction with childbirth, fewer incidences of postpartum depression, increased self-esteem, better mother-infant interaction, and improved breastfeeding success. A birth coach will stay with you during your labor until your baby is about an hour old, in addition to a few prenatal visits and one postnatal visit. Birth coaching services can range from pro bono to $3,000. Most labor support coaches charge between $500 and $2,000, depending on experience and certification. You can get labor coach recommendations at maternity centers, OB/GYN offices, yoga studio community boards, via DONA International, and on websites like www.thebump.com.

You want to make sure you feel a level of chemistry, comfort, and safety with your coach, as she will accompany you during one of the most intimate and eventful experiences of your life. Whatever you do, go with your gut. If you meet a prospective coach and you're not sure about her, keep looking. You can trust your inner diva on this one! Use the following questions to see if this person is right for you and your family:

- What inspired you to enter this field of work?
- What certifications do you hold?
- How long have you been a doula and how many births have you attended?
- What types of births have you attended—home birth, hospital, birth center?
- How do I get in touch with you when labor begins—are you always on call? When and where will you join me?
- If you are unavailable when I go into labor, do you have backups?
- What is your philosophy on childbirth? (Make sure your birth preferences are compatible with her practices and beliefs.)
- What techniques will you use to help me move through labor?
- How long will you stay with me after labor?
- What happens if I need a C-section?

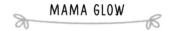

- Do you provide postpartum services? Do you have experience helping nursing mothers?

- What's your fee and refund policy? What does it cover?

For more info on labor support coaches/doulas, please check out DONA International, the certifying body for women who provide labor support, at www .dona.org.

Tips for the Home Stretch

You're so close to meeting your baby, the last thing you may be thinking about is going on a date with your partner, husband, or boyfriend. But if this is your first child, these are some of the last days you will have alone with your sweetie. Take advantage of these quiet moments. Plan things you love to do but never make time for, like checking out a play, baking, getting massages or acupuncture, or taking a day trip to the beach. Mama Glow Icon and fashion designer Rachel Roy says she spent this time catching up on reading, particularly texts that explore other cultures. Let's not forget to continually massage your belly and low-back areas with a quality oil or cream, as discussed in the second-trimester chapters.

Eat small meals throughout the day. This will help you to stay energized and will regulate your blood sugar. Make sure the meals are loaded up with glow foods! Pack on the protein, extra calcium, iron, and potassium, in addition to your daily prenatal vitamin. Remember, your baby is putting on a lot of weight in these last few weeks of pregnancy—about half a pound per week—so make sure she's getting the nourishment she needs.

Before you deliver, it's a great idea to take a breastfeeding class or check out a meeting at La Leche League, an international breastfeeding support organization. You can find out more at www.lalecheleague.org. The more you know about breastfeeding, the more confident you will be when the day arrives. These classes will teach proper latching techniques and various ways to hold your baby to your breast. Most important, they will provide you with resources for support, including lactation consultants and breastfeeding support groups. While you're at it, contact local pediatricians and find one whose practices are aligned with your beliefs and who makes you feel at ease. Get recommendations from friends and health-care providers, and search databases online.

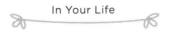

Let's Talk About Sex

Once you are at about 37 weeks you can start taking evening primrose oil to help "ripen" your cervix. This oil is full of prostaglandins, which turn a hard and rigid cervix into a soft and squishy one. Think of it like a hard peach that ripens and becomes soft and mushy—that's exactly what your cervix is going to do! The oil comes in capsules or cold-pressed in a bottle. The oil can be taken three times daily for up to ten days. If you haven't gone into labor by then you can stop taking the oil.

Another great way to ripen the cervix? Have sex! Yup, I said it, ladies. Semen deposits against the cervix help it to ripen because semen also contains prostaglandins! Isn't Mother Nature clever? The more good sex you have leading up to delivery, the more relaxed your pelvic floor muscles will be for labor. Sounds like a pretty good deal to me.

Sex also promotes oxytocin production. Oxytocin is the "love hormone"—or "love juice"—which is coursing through your system at high-level arousal and peaking at climax. But it's also the mothering hormone, so it's produced in copious amounts during labor, peaking at birth.

So if you've been having some good lovin' these last few months of pregnancy, not only have you been having a lot of fun, you've been igniting your pleasure pathways and increasing your chances of having a pleasurable birth. If you haven't been in the mood, that's fine, too. Many women experience low sex drive during pregnancy, for a combination of reasons. These may include low self-image, not feeling sexy, not feeling in control, feeling tired or uncomfortable, lifestyle factors, or just feeling *huge*.

If you've found yourself in this boat during pregnancy, then evening primrose oil is for you. An added bonus is that this oil contains essential fatty acids and helps to make the tissues more elastic, preventing tearing of the perineum during labor. This is great news, since you'll be doing lots of stretching to push your baby out.

Get Comfy Cozy

Comfort is a big deal during labor. It's a workout, and you're going to need stamina and support to get through it. Practicing comfort measures, postures, and coping techniques with your birth partner will help him or her better serve you in the last weeks of pregnancy—and during labor as well. Counterpressure using the heel of the hands and pressing into either side of the sacrum is a lifesaver when

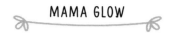
you are experiencing intense sensation during contractions. Touch transmits intention very powerfully, so having a birth partner who knows how you like to be touched is really helpful when moving through the final stretch. For instructional videos please visit www.mamaglow.com.

Sister Circle

Defining your sister circle and identifying support systems for pregnancy and birth is critical now. It's important to build a strong network of cheerleaders so you are not alone. Nothing is sustainable without community. Surround yourself with people who are smarter than you are, and who have the skills and resources to help support you. This will ensure that you thrive in this third trimester and beyond.

Make yourself at home with your sister circle. If you don't have a support group you can start by connecting with women who have shared interests—in your book club, or dance or yoga class. Ask questions of mothers around you, and gather resources. Call on your starting lineup of wonder women to come help out at your home prior to the birth so you can relax and don't have so much to do on your own. Choose a mixed group of women, including seasoned mamas and single friends. Variety is key here for a few reasons. First, veteran moms know exactly how to make themselves useful, are often efficient, and usually know their way around the kitchen, so meals will be taken care of. Your single girlfriends, on the other hand, can run errands, grocery shop, answer phones, help clean, and hold the baby to give you a few minutes to take a shower! Get your circle ready before your baby comes so you're not phoning and texting friends in search of support when you need it most.

Ask one of your closest friends to help coordinate a rotation of women—you don't want all your helpers at the house at the same time! You'll want to have your support staggered so you can best utilize your team. Not to mention that you'll want some bonding time with your new baby. Designate duties ahead of time, based on each person's strengths.

An interesting thing I learned about this transformative experience of becoming a mother was that not all my friends were ready for me to become a new person. Not all of them knew how to grow with me and support me on my journey. Subsequently, as I moved into motherhood I lost some of my former friends in the process. But there is always loss involved in personal growth—you have to let go of attachment to who you used to be, which may include letting go of some of your old friends. You're moving into the new you, so surround yourself with the

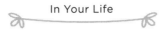

best people—those who are 100 percent ready and willing to support you during this critical time.

Birth Bag Basics

Be prepared, and pack your birth bag—your travel case—in advance. Even if you are birthing at home, it's nice to have a packed bag on hand, just in case you need to travel to the hospital for any unforeseen reason. I had my birth bag ready for weeks! I thought it was the coolest thing to be packing for my trip to the birth center, a whopping nine blocks away. I packed things like essential oils, music, comfy socks, a yoga mat, receiving blankets, menstrual pads, and witch hazel (which is a must for a vaginal birth—see the Birth Bag Must-Haves List on the next page for details). If you are birthing in a hospital setting, keep in mind that you might want to bring your own clothes. It makes you feel more comfortable and at home to wear your own things, rather than a hospital gown. That said, hospital gowns are available for your use in the fashionable open-back smock style if that tickles your fancy.

Birth can be messy, of course, so if you do choose to wear your own duds, be prepared to have them soiled afterward. Hospitals can also be on the chilly side, so having a few sweaters and socks, as well as bringing your own blanket, is a good idea. Of course you want to consider what the baby will wear home! Bring a beanie cap, newborn gown, receiving blankets, and diapers. There are some great eco-friendly diapers on the market now, including Seventh Generation and G-Diapers. Good old-fashioned cloth is always a great option as well. My mother cloth-diapered both my sister and me back in the '80s, and I still admire her for that.

Most important, make sure you have adequate food and drink with you. Labor is serious work, the hardest work for the best payoff. But it doesn't come without a huge expenditure of energy. It's best to have food and drink on hand so you can stay well nourished. I like to bring energy bars, almonds, fresh fruit, and smoothies when I attend births. I find it easier for the mothers to nosh on snacks than to deal with a fork and knife to eat. Also, bring plant-based protein-rich foods to help replace the drained energy stores. The complex carbs found in fruits and veggies will convert into readily usable energy—which you'll be grateful for when you've been laboring for a while and it's almost time to push. I'm a big fan of smoothies and soups, which can both be sipped through a straw. They ensure you stay well hydrated and keep passing urine.

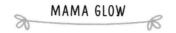

Birth Bag Must-Haves List

What else do you need in your travel case? Here's a complete list of birth bag must-haves. I recommended that you pack your bag by week 33, which allows you to get ready for showtime, just in case your baby decides to make an early appearance.

- ☐ *Cozy Socks.* Bring at least two pairs. Get ones with traction on the soles to keep from sliding on slick floors.

- ☐ *Sweater.* Preferably a wrap, button-down, or loose pull-over.

- ☐ *Maternity Bras.* Bring two, plus nursing pads.

- ☐ *Sweatpants.* I'm not a fan of sweat suits unless you are running up and down a soccer field for a living, but after labor they can be very comfy.

- ☐ *Hair Bands.* Don't forget headbands, hair clips, or ponytail holders to secure your hair.

- ☐ *Toiletries.* Toothbrush, toothpaste, deodorant.

- ☐ *Lip Balm.* Hospitals can be very dry.

- ☐ *Camera.* Don't forget an extra memory card and charger!

- ☐ *Cell Phone.* Draw up a contact list for who you want to call after the birth.

- ☐ *Paperwork.* Bring insurance forms, hospital forms, and your birth preferences sheet.

- ☐ *Going-Home Clothes.* For you, include flat shoes! For baby, include beanie cap, outfit, and receiving blankets.

- ☐ *Pantry-on-the-Go.* Make sure to pack your go-to glow foods to keep nourished during labor. (See some of my suggestions in the previous section.)

- ☐ *Music.* CDs or iPod and dock with speakers.

- ☐ *Labor Mate Phone App.* Labor Mate is a contraction timer available for the iPhone, iTouch, and Android devices. It makes it much easier to keep track of the contractions. Download through iTunes for 99 cents. If you don't have a smartphone device, use a stopwatch and notepad to keep track.

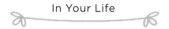
☐ *Essential Oils.* Using essential oils during labor is a wonderful way to help center and relax. The oils work on the primal brain, helping to keep you in an altered brain-wave state. You'll want to use high-quality oils like the Young Living brand. Excellent oils to have on hand include geranium, jasmine, neroli, lavender, rose, and myrrh.

☐ *Mood Items.* Bring pictures, icons, and anything that makes you feel at home. Pictures of family members, nature, inspiring quotes, or objects will personalize your birthing space.

☐ *Artificial Candles.* Soft light sources create a moody space. These battery-operated candles are a great, safe, hospital-approved alternative to real candles.

☐ *Push Presents.* This is for your birth partner, not you, to bring. It's a gift that your birth partner gives you at the time of pushing. With roots in East Indian tradition, gifting to celebrate birthing women became popular in the U.S. in the early '90s.

☐ *Witch-Hazel Pads.* These pads help soothe the vulva and perineal tissues after vaginal birth. You can make your own by dousing thick maxi pads with witch hazel and popping in the freezer. (You'll thank me for this one.)

Soundscape

What sounds do you want present at your labor? What song, if any, might you want to play once your baby arrives? My son's father had a very popular radio show and made extraordinary mix CDs for my labor. I had this grand plan to play music throughout the labor. Now mind you, this was before everybody had iPods. I ended up not using the music until my son arrived. He was very calm and relaxed at birth. As soon as he decided to have his first cry, his father walked over to the CD player and inserted Erik Satie's *Gymnopédies*—a recording that I often listened to in order to relax before bed while pregnant. Suddenly Fulano—not even a full hour old—fell silent. I like to think he was mesmerized by the sound he was hearing for the first time without the aqua barrier!

Play music for your baby, but also for yourself. Gather some playlists of inspiring music and sounds that will take you into a sacred space while birthing, should you choose to use it. Be sure to vary the types of music on your playlists.

Instrumentals and ambient music work well, as do natural sounds like the sea crashing against the shore and mantra chanting. You're going to need very different sounds for early labor than you will for transition—when it's time to push—so make sure you have some more motivational music for the big moment.

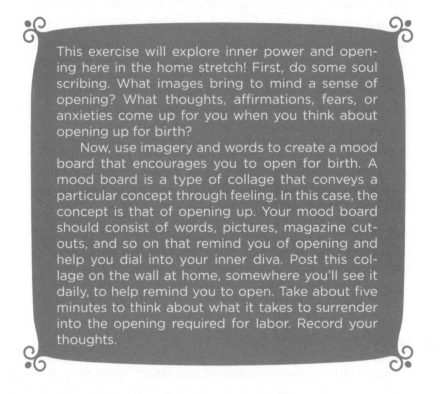

This exercise will explore inner power and opening here in the home stretch! First, do some soul scribing. What images bring to mind a sense of opening? What thoughts, affirmations, fears, or anxieties come up for you when you think about opening up for birth?

Now, use imagery and words to create a mood board that encourages you to open for birth. A mood board is a type of collage that conveys a particular concept through feeling. In this case, the concept is that of opening up. Your mood board should consist of words, pictures, magazine cutouts, and so on that remind you of opening and help you dial into your inner diva. Post this collage on the wall at home, somewhere you'll see it daily, to help remind you to open. Take about five minutes to think about what it takes to surrender into the opening required for labor. Record your thoughts.

Blissful Birth and Cocktail Party

Birth is a dance. Along the way a cocktail of hormones will cascade into your bloodstream and produce an effect that is masterfully designed to make you and your baby fall in love. Our culture views birth as a violent, painful, and disempowering experience. For generations women have taken a back seat when it comes to childbirth, allowing modern obstetrics to push a technocratic birth model that has little respect for the power of the female body, and now it's time to reclaim our bodies as sacred sites and to trust our inner divas who know exactly how to give birth. I know birth to be a potent experience that reshaped my life, that gave me a power center that I still stand from today. The cocktail of hormones formulated

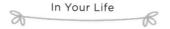

by the goddess herself is designed to carry you through to the other side, making you feel so good that you'd do it again and again.

The Hormones of Labor

Most people don't realize how complex the birth process is and yet how innately equipped we are to undergo it. There are some important hormones you should know about as you prepare for labor. Maybe you'll get some cool points in your birthing class if you reference these.

Oxytocin—What's Not to Love?

We've talked about this one before. But did you know that in addition to being a bonding hormone, oxytocin is the hormone that starts your uterine contractions? At the onset of labor, your body produces copious amounts of this hormone. Mothers who are induced into labor are given Pitocin, a synthetic form of oxytocin. Unfortunately, Pitocin interferes with the release of oxytocin from the brain. In that way it disrupts the primal rhythmic pattern of contractions—a gradual movement of waves through the body—and replaces it with an aggressive climb toward more intense contractions. The intensity can cause both mom and baby unnecessary distress. Best to avoid Pitocin if possible, and stick to your natural oxytocin.

Not only does oxytocin start uterine contractions, but it also helps to stop postpartum hemorrhage. What's more, oxytocin continues to be secreted when your baby suckles at the breast, and since there is a hardwired connection between the breasts and the uterus, the suckling stimulates the uterus to contract back to its normal size. And again, it helps you to bond and communicate through love with this tiny new family member.

PEA: Obsessed with Phenylethylamine

If oxytocin is the love hormone, then PEA is the *falling in love* hormone. You might be surprised to hear that this birth hormone is also found in elevated amounts in the brains of folks with obsessive compulsive disorder. Why would it be biologically advantageous to equip us with such a hormone? People with OCD are overly attentive to—even obsessed with—a particular set of triggers. Mother Nature, in her infinite wisdom, knew exactly what she was doing when she put

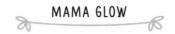

this hormone into the labor mix. She wants us to be obsessed with our babies, to pay attention to every little detail. Unfortunately, we only get to experience this hormone when we go through the primal journey to birth—interventions get in the way. Medicine can disconnect the mind-body experience, meaning this delicious hormone isn't secreted.

Dimethyltryptamine (DMT): The God Chemical

Called "the God chemical," DMT is a psychedelic substance produced by your pineal gland. DMT is found naturally in various sources, and is related to human neurotransmitters such as serotonin and melatonin. People all around the globe travel to visit shamans for guided ceremony with the indigenous psychedelics Ayahuasca and peyote, both of which contain DMT. So much work, just to get the blissful experience that your female body naturally creates at birth! This "God chemical" naturally peaks at birth, and also gets released during orgasm and when you die. I call this chemical "The Big Bang," because it shows up at the three major portals of life: birth, procreation, and death. It's also released in smaller amounts just as you enter REM sleep, as well as during lucid dreaming and meditation. DMT is first produced by the human fetus on the 49th day of development, according to Dr. Rick Strassman, who specializes in psychiatry and has conducted extensive studies on the effects of DMT. Meaning as early as the first trimester, your little one is already experiencing God.

Endorphins: Natural Opiates

Finally, the body's natural opiates are proteins released during labor—locking into receptors that might otherwise feel pain, they act as an analgesic. In its place, you experience intense, arousing sensation. Thresholds of pain and arousal change as you move through your labor. Beta-endorphins have a numbing effect on par with morphine. Research shows that women begin to release endorphins prior to labor.

Fear and Anxiety (a.k.a. Birth Kryptonite)

So fear is not your friend. Please say that a few times out loud right now so you get it through your head. (Go on. I'll wait.) Fear is the antidote to a wonderful

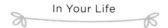
cocktail of hormones and natural substances that are working with you to birth your baby. When you become afraid of the pain, of needles, of a C-section, for the baby's safety, you release cortisol—the direct antagonist to birth hormones. It literally turns off your cocktail service; oxytocin comes to a halt. Just as you can't orgasm during sex if you're anxious, afraid, or stressed out, birth is not going to go according to your plans if you are hanging on to a lot of fear.

Anxiety is the stepchild of fear. The best way to get back on track when you start to get fearful is to breathe and connect to affirming thoughts—it's that simple.

I am powerful now and the universe supports me and my baby.
I have everything I need inside to birth my baby.
I open my body to the miracle of new life.

We lose control of our fluid yin goddess energy when we become fearful. You can be in love or in fear—you choose what you want most for your baby.

F.E.A.R. = F@$K Everything and Run

On a spiritual level, fear dials you into the pain cycle. You want to be in the *love cycle*! That's the energetic space in which you created your baby in the first place. Fear makes us forget our power. Dr. Grantly Dick-Read in his research in the 1930s theorized that the more a laboring woman feared the process, the tenser her body would become and the more pain she would feel during labor. When you experience fear, your body releases chemicals to help you respond to the perceived threat and escape the danger, whether real or imaginary. This response, generally known as the fight-or-flight response, causes the blood to rush away from your internal organs toward your head and limbs, where it can help give you the strength, speed, and wits necessary to get away safely. Fight-or-flight robs your uterus of the oxygen it needs to perform rhythmic contractions.

Often when fear arises, labor actually halts. It's a biological mechanism to preserve mom and baby. Imagine an ancestor mammal mama laboring in the wild. She would secure a safe place, tucked away from the elements, and begin the process of labor. If she sensed a predator looming about, suddenly her brain would cease to produce the birthing hormones. In an instant, cortisol and adrenaline would take their place—flooding the system. She'd take flight to get to safety. Once in a secure location the stress hormones would wear off again. Her shallow breathing would slow and labor would resume.

The fear, tension, and pain actually stop labor from progressing. The muscles that open the cervix contract instead of relaxing. The result is painful labor, where your muscles are working against the grain. They have access to very little oxygen, so the cramping factor is high. When you are afraid, your sphincters shut tight. If you aren't relaxed, your pelvic floor, uterine muscles, cervix, and surrounding sphincters will close off—halting the labor for the time being until you can get back to a place of calm.

Unlike animals in the wild, we think our way into fear by creating what-if scenarios in our heads. We don't even need a real threat to initiate a fight-or-flight response in the body. Fearful thoughts or a stressful set of circumstances will do just fine. Given our high-speed, busy lives, many women initiate labor in states of high stress.

The pain a laboring woman experiences as a result of stress and anxiety only serves to affirm her deepest, darkest fears about her body and the birth process: that labor is an excruciating experience and that her body is incapable of handling the pain that lies ahead. She begins to cycle into more fearful thoughts, which tense her up more—leading to only more pain. The cycle goes on and on like this until there is a conscious break. The break comes if and when you realize that *you* are the one creating the pain—and that you can also bring about your pleasure. I'm not saying labor is a walk in the park—but it doesn't have to be a dreadful experience by any means. We can manage how we experience the pain, which can be intense. If we accept that pain will be present, when it comes, we can focus on its purpose. You will notice each contraction and how it grows to a peak, where you experience the full edge of sensation, and when it comes down. Consider that each wave has a purpose—to guide your baby down and out of your body. With each contraction you are a baby step closer to meeting your newborn.

The first step toward reestablishing the connection to the primal experience is to recognize that you are saying the "FEAR" mantra (Fuck Everything and Run). At that point you can stop yourself from trying to flee your birth (which you can't actually escape—sorry, honey). Just noticing you're in fear is like hitting ctrl-alt-delete on your computer. It's a spiritual reboot, and guess what? Love is your operating system. It's that love energy that made your baby and that loving energy will guide your baby out of your womb and into the world.

When you stay in connection with your inner glow—your goddess guru—you will more easily trust your body and the divinity of the process. Then you can allow sweet surrender. Your inner diva will show you the way. Your energy will go wherever you send it. It is obedient. My advice is to simply stay in the glow zone.

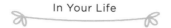
Transmute any form of anxiety through deep breathing, movement meditations, and visualizations to help you stay in the flow. Primal movements include hip swivels, swaying on hands and knees, sitting with legs crossed while moving the pelvis in circles, and so on.

Courage is feeling the fear and doing it anyway. When we *encourage,* we help others to find space to move beyond fear. That's my job here. I want you to have a different dialogue with your body, one that says:

> *I trust and honor you.*
> *We can do this.*
> *I was made with everything I need to do this.*

Stand and Deliver

A baby learns whether the earth is a safe place within the first day of life. How you are born is very important. There is so much focus on palliative care and quality of life for the dying, as there should be, but the same attention should be placed on how a baby comes into the world and how a mother is born into the role of caretaker. She should be respected and treated as a client, not a patient—there *is* a difference. How do we establish a normal birth process? It starts with knowing your options and knowing what is the normal course of labor and believing in it—practicing like you've done all these months, standing up for what you want and deserve, and delivering on your terms. That's what I mean by stand and deliver: get off your back and show them how it's done!

Free to Be! Movement During Labor

A woman has to be given the right to move instinctively. In a home birth and birth center this is encouraged, but not as much in hospitals. If a woman is in bed during her labor, she loses the advantage of having gravity on her side. And two common birthing strategies, continuous electronic fetal monitoring (EFM) and epidural anesthesia, keep you lying on your back. To get moving while in labor, try the following:

- Request intermittent monitoring versus continuous—it's fine as long as you're not high risk.

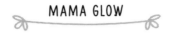
- Try all noninvasive pain management strategies first: a massage, counterpressure, shower or bath, vibrator, changes in position, pressure points.

- Use a birthing ball to move and swivel your hips and try walking to increase the contractions if they slow down.

Optimal Positions for Birth

Pain is purposeful. It guides you instinctively into the movements and positions that make you more comfortable and help the baby navigate your pelvis. When an epidural is introduced, that feedback mechanism is lost and you are no longer aware of what is happening below your waist. When you are upright in a squat, your pelvis is 30 percent more open. Hello! That is major, considering what you are about to push through, honey. To avoid the supine, lying-on-your-back position, try the following:

- During pregnancy, spend time in positions that help the baby position itself correctly. These include Child's Pose, hands and knees (Cat and Cow), sitting forward in a chair with your spine nice and tall, sitting cross-legged, or squatting.

- Avoid an epidural or other interventions that would render you immobile, and enlist a skilled birth coach for your support team to help you try to find more comfortable positions.

- Ask for a squat bar, which fits right onto your bed and helps women to assume a more upright position during the pushing stage.

- Try the side-lying squat position. This is a favorable way to rest and try the first few pushes when it's time to deliver.

A Labor of Love

Time to review the anatomy of labor and birth using the prenatal yoga principles. Get acquainted with the hormones—you're being tested on this stuff! At the end of the first stage of labor, the cervix is dilated to 10 centimeters. In mothers having their first child, this stage usually lasts 12 to 16 hours. For women having subsequent children, the first stage lasts around 6 to 7 hours. That said, I have seen

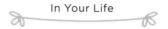

first-timers with lightning-speed deliveries. You just never know . . . but that's the beauty of it. I was at a labor that took five days and luckily my backup doula and I could divide the time. This mom was headstrong and determined to have a natural birth, and ended up with every intervention possible. I also attended a labor where a first-time mom called me at the onset of her contractions and her labor moved so quickly that she was already pushing when I met her at the hospital, and she delivered in triage.

Early Labor

Your baby sends a signal that she is ready to be born by producing oxytocin and sending it to your brain. Your brain then signals your uterus to start contracting. During the early or latent phase, the cervix dilates to 4 centimeters. The duration of the first phase is the longest, averaging around eight hours. Your contractions may be irregular, progressing to rhythmic and methodical. The sensation you feel at this early stage may be similar to menstrual cramping: aching, fullness, and backache. You may feel mild or intense sensation—everyone is different. You will still be able to walk freely and walking is usually more comfortable than sitting as it moves the pubic bones and opens the pelvis. Most women spend these hours at home, since home is where labor tends to progress most quickly. You'll be more comfortable in your own personal space. At this point you are setting an *intention* to stay calm, centered, and focused. You may feel eager, excited, and social—wanting to call your family and friends—but try to get some rest instead. You've got a big day ahead. At this point you are practicing *mindfulness*. It is important that you conserve your energy for the work of labor, not wasting it on mind-chatter and fear. At this point *do* call your health-care provider, labor support coach, and anyone else on your birth team.

Active Labor

Active labor is marked by regular contractions that become longer, stronger, and closer together over time. Most providers recommend that you go to the hospital or birthing center when your contractions are four minutes apart, last more than one minute, and have been under way for at least one hour. This is the 411 principle.

If you're birthing at home, your midwife should have arrived by now. You and your birth partner should be measuring your contractions from the start of one contraction to the beginning of the next. Try using the Labor Mate phone app, which I mentioned on page 192. It's a mere 99 cents and well worth it.

When you are in active labor, your labor partner's support is crucial. Touch, holding, caressing, massage, and silence are all helpful. The waves of contractions are growing stronger, longer, and closer together. You are in a rhythm. Continue to use your tools of visioning, breathing, and movement. You are *tuning in.*

Contractions will be about three to four minutes apart, lasting 40 to 60 seconds. You may have a tightening feeling in your pubic area and increasing pressure in your back. It's critical to remember that you are *flexible* and you can get into optimal positioning for your comfort and your baby's descent. Your body will indicate what is most comfortable, and your birth coach will offer positions as well.

Transition

Transition is the most challenging phase of labor and also the shortest, lasting from 30 minutes to two hours. The cervix is opening the last few centimeters, from 7 to 10 centimeters. The sensations may be intense, as the cervix stretches and the baby descends into the birth canal. All of your energy is now concentrated on doing the work of labor. Try to remain calm and focused as your uterus does what it knows how to do. You are *opening.* At the end of transition, you may feel a strong urge to push the baby out. The baby is ready to be born.

During the second stage of labor, the highest levels of oxytocin are flooding your bloodstream. The baby's head stretches your vagina and perineum. Your practitioner may begin to massage and stretch the vulva and perineum using evening primrose, almond, or jojoba oil. The pressure may feel like you have to poop; the urge to push, or bear down, may be fierce. But follow your practitioner's instruction, as pushing too early will cause the cervix to become swollen.

It's also very important to push *with your breath*. Otherwise you'll experience the phenomenon of "purple pushing"—pushing until your face turns purple, which restricts oxygen flow to you and your baby. Remember, your breath is your freedom. Take a few breaths during that push period and bear down, easing the baby out. As soon as the widest part of the baby's head appears at the vaginal opening, we say the baby has crowned. Stay focused, diva: in the next few pushes, your baby will be born.

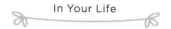

As soon as the baby is out, your body starts to reward you for your focused effort. DMT, the "God chemical" we talked about, is being released by your pineal gland. Endorphins are swirling all about. You'll feel completely blissful as you hold your baby for the first time, experiencing total *glow power.*

After Birth

Contractions may stop for a while, then resume in order to deliver the placenta. The delivery of the placenta is the shortest stage of the birth cycle, lasting from 5 to 15 minutes. It's also the least eventful for most women, perhaps because they are so occupied having their new child in their arms!

Speaking of which, your baby is probably looking to suckle. Breastfeeding stimulates oxytocin production, which helps to contract the uterus back down to its normal size and stop bleeding. It also helps the placenta detach from the uterine wall spontaneously. If the baby stays attached to the cord she will instinctively climb up to the nipple. So there really isn't any reason in rushing a placenta from detaching or cutting the cord right away. Research shows a two-minute delay in cord clamping increases a baby's iron reserve by 27 to 47 mg, which is equivalent to one to two months of an infant's iron requirements. This could help to prevent iron deficiency from developing before six months of age. You can express to your birth practitioner that you would like to allow your body the time to naturally deliver the placenta as well as delay in cutting the cord.

You will be observed closely for the next few hours to make certain that your uterus is contracting properly and bleeding is not excessive. Take this time to rest and get acquainted with your new baby. Now's the time to emanate *gratitude.*

The journey I just described is a typical birth that is not interrupted by intervention. When you take the biochemical, neurological journey and experience that total oneness, ecstasy, and bliss, you're riding the Mama Glow! It's *your* cocktail party, mama, designed to make you fall madly in love with your baby, an important survival and bonding strategy. The gratitude you feel when holding your baby for the first time is inexplicable.

Planning for the Unplanned

Sometimes things don't go as planned, and you and your baby may have a different outcome than you first envisioned—that's okay. The goal is a healthy and

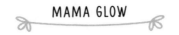

happy bundle of joy, so act from a place of nonjudgment. When you are in the glow zone it doesn't matter if your baby comes in a different way. Remember, birth is not a competition. So it's best to plan for the unplanned, and learn how you can help prevent some of these outcomes that may not be your choice for birth.

Ins and Outs of Induction

In 2002, 20.6 percent of labors were induced. By 2007, inductions nearly doubled—mostly for nonmedical reasons. The rise in labor induction is directly correlated to the rise in cesarean sections, because induction can put both mother and baby in distress. Consider the following alternatives to clinical induction:

- Practice patience. A 2002 study showed a median pregnancy length of 41 weeks plus one day in women who had never given birth before, and a 40-week, 3-day average pregnancy length in mothers going for their second or third baby. Medical inductions are usually necessary after 42 weeks because of an increased risk of stillbirth (caused by a decreased flow of oxygen and nutrients through the placenta).

- Get your hormones naturally. You already know all about prostaglandin, which is found in many cervix-ripening drugs. But remember, it is also naturally found in semen and evening primrose oil. Then there's oxytocin, which is used to induce labor. It is naturally produced during orgasm and nipple stimulation. In other words, a good ole romp around the bedroom can get things going in lieu of using drugs.

- Strip the membranes. Your physician or midwife can swipe your cervical membranes during an internal exam. She'll use a finger to swipe against the cervix; for some, it initiates labor within a few days.

- Try ancient secrets. Castor oil, black and blue cohosh, and acupuncture have all been used for centuries to naturally induce labor. Check with your practitioner team to decide what would be best for you.

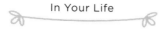

C-Section

Cesarean section is an intervention that is on the rise—from about 5 percent in 1970 to more than 30 percent today. There are instances where this procedure will save the life of the mother and child. But in many cases it is done out of convenience. I like to call it an unnecessarian-section. By the time a woman has been induced, given an epidural, and labored on her back, it's almost too late for anything but a surgical outcome. Hoping to avoid a C-section? Try these tips:

- Avoid interventions that put you at higher risk for a C-section, especially an induction (unless it is medically necessary). If you are attempting a vaginal birth after a previous cesarean section, you absolutely should not be induced since it can increase your risk of uterine rupture.

- Labor at home for as long as comfortable. The later you go to your birthing place, the less likely you are to be faced with unnecessary interventions. I stay home with my laboring clients until they are experiencing contractions at least four minutes apart and lasting about a minute.

- A poorly positioned baby is cited as the reason for a C-section in about 25 percent of cases. Some undesirable positions include babies in breech presentation, transverse, sideways, or posterior, meaning your baby's spine is next to your spine. Some exercises encouraging an optimal fetal position (OFP) include practicing squatting, taking regular breaks to walk around if you do a lot of sitting, washing the floors on all fours, placing a cushion under your hips to tilt your pelvis forward when sitting down, and watching television while resting forward over a birthing ball. These simple lifestyle adjustments will help move your baby into an anterior position.

Episiotomy

Studies suggest that births assisted by midwives are five times less likely to involve episiotomies than those handled by obstetricians. An episiotomy is the surgical cutting of the tissue between the vagina and the anus. The procedure is supposed to ease difficult deliveries, but it can result in more severe tearing, blood

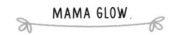

loss, infection, urinary and fecal incontinence, and painful intercourse. There is major erectile tissue that physicians cut through without regard to the effect it may have on a mother postpartum.

To avoid an episiotomy, work with a midwife. Or, be sure your physician knows you do not want an episiotomy unless a true medical emergency warrants it. To naturally avoid tearing during delivery, try the following:

- It takes time for the perineum to stretch, so try laboring upright as much as possible. That way you let gravity work in your favor.

- Ask your birth attendant to hold the baby's head so that it slowly and gradually eases through the vaginal opening.

- Ask your practitioner to use almond or jojoba oil to massage and stretch the vulva and perineal tissues as the baby is descending.

> *Glow Tip: Perineal massage at the end of pregnancy and during labor can help stretch and prepare the perineum for delivery. I've never tried it myself, and it works for some and not others. But what I know for sure is that you can stretch to accommodate your baby's head. If you do tear, it is usually only a surface tear versus a deep cut into the erectile structure of the perineum.*

There are emergency cases in which these interventions are necessary. If you are faced with such a situation, keep in mind that a healthy baby and mommy are most important. My hope is for you to be prepared with information and options to make decisions that are right for you.

P.U.S.H.: Pray Until Something Happens

Push is a four-letter word. Debra Pascali-Bonaro, founding board member of DONA International, says you should never yell four-letter words at a laboring woman! In other words, no yelling, "Push!" Pushing is a natural urge that you will feel without needing to be reminded.

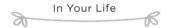

I want to flip the focus here to another type of pushing, and that is one of perseverance with *prayer*. So while the goddess is working through you to birth this new life, if you find yourself at a moment where you need to call upon a higher power, you can close your eyes and pray. Prayer is when we make a petition, asking for exactly what we need in the moment we need it. It can be followed by meditation, which is when we listen for guidance. So in the moment when you feel overwhelmed, like you can't do it, know that the sensation can never overcome you. The sensation *is* you—it's your own glow that's been contained inside you all this time. Nature and our bodies are always communicating with us. We've just forgotten how to listen. So trust and move into the unknown; that's where magic happens.

No Separation of the Mother and Baby Dyad

Immediately following birth, a healthy baby should be placed skin-to-skin on the mother's abdomen or chest. The baby should be able to feel and smell you, mommy. From your belly the baby can be dried, covered with warm blankets, and allowed to do "the crawl" to your breast to begin breastfeeding. Once the baby latches to your breast, uterine contractions begin to help reduce postpartum bleeding. To avoid separation, try the following:

- Allow the cord to stay intact until it ceases pulsation, then clamp and cut with the baby on your chest.

- Avoid a planned C-section (an "unnecessarian") and limit interventions, which could lead to complications and require mother or baby to receive special treatment postpartum.

- Make sure your provider and the hospital have a copy of your birth plan, which includes your postpartum and newborn care expectations.

- Delay or waive any tests or procedures that aren't necessary right away. Opt out of any optional procedures you prefer to avoid altogether.

- You can go against hospital policy, but you may need to sign a waiver for legal purposes. If you don't feel in control and feel forced to stick to policy, consider birthing elsewhere.

Mama Glow Checklist:

Use this checklist to help remember everything you want to do before the big day. Take a moment to see what you need to prioritize in preparation for your blissful birth.

- ☐ Create your birth plan (vision).
- ☐ Secure a labor support coach for labor and/or postnatal support.
- ☐ Schedule a personal date with yourself and your partner.
- ☐ Continue to massage the belly, hips, and low back with belly oil or cream.
- ☐ Eat multiple small meals throughout the day to keep balanced blood sugar and prevent heartburn.
- ☐ Fortify your diet with adequate iron, protein, calcium, and potassium.
- ☐ Take evening primrose oil to ripen the cervix (or if you have a partner and he's a guy, have sex—semen is full of prostaglandins).
- ☐ Attend a breastfeeding class or La Leche League meeting.
- ☐ Find a great pediatrician.
- ☐ Practice birth positions and coping techniques.
- ☐ Call on your sister circle to prep meals for after the birth and to help with household chores.
- ☐ Pack your birth bag.
- ☐ Make playlists for your birth.

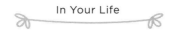

Glow Tips for the Home Stretch

Haley Binn, writer, eco-lover, health advocate, volunteer, and mother, is a Mama Glow Icon because she balances self-care in pregnancy while raising a family. Haley prioritizes family yet still manages to have time alone to engage in activities that feed her soul. Haley shares her glow tips for the final days of pregnancy:

- *Relish Your Quiet Moments.* These won't last forever. My goal in pregnancy is to always stay in the moment. This is the time for preparation and rest is a big part of that.

- *Get a Blow Out.* Have your hair done: let the stylist shampoo and massage your scalp and style your hair, not to look good for the staff at your birth but for *you* to feel regal and look fabulous for you alone.

You should pat yourself on the back, girlfriend. This has been an amazing ride. Not only do you have the extraordinary opportunity to give birth, but you, too, are birthed as a mother. We still have one stop more to go on this journey. Our next section takes you into your new life postpartum with your baby. You'll learn how to eat for breastfeeding and explore what I call "boob foods." You will be introduced to your postnatal yoga practice and learn helpful tips for adjusting to your new life with your baby bundle.

part V

WELLNESS A.D.
(AFTER DELIVERY)

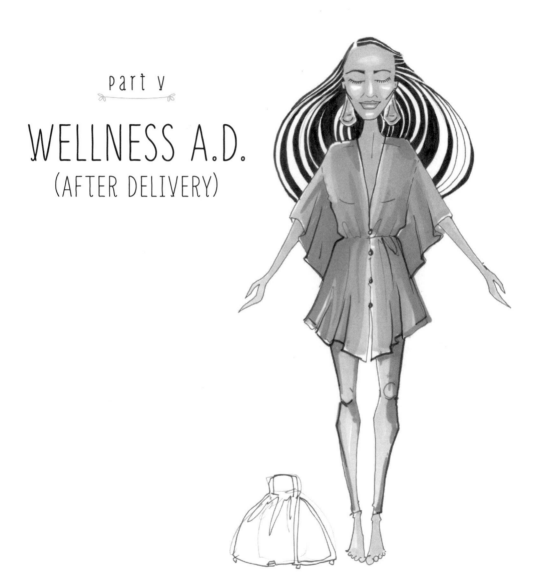

CHAPTER 17

POSTPARTUM AND MAMA-GLOW MOJO

Groovin' Your New Abundant Life

Congratulations, mama, you did it! It's been an amazing journey, full of growth on so many levels. Now the real fun starts: bonding with your baby, managing a new life with your bundle of joy, and getting back on track to a lean, mean, and brand-new post-baby body. There are many interesting challenges ahead, but you've already made it through the biggest rite of passage and blessing of your life: pregnancy, labor, and delivery. It's been a pleasure guiding you along the way. I hope you enjoyed the wild ride.

Now it's time to talk about changes in your body, feelings you may be having, mood swings, euphoria, and baby blues. I'll reassure you about discomforts including tender breasts, engorgement, and weak pelvic floor muscles—as well as hormonal shifts, exhaustion, low sex drive, and low milk production. We'll talk about calling in support to help you thrive through this period, and how long it should last. We'll explore all the postpartum delights from the ever-popular baby-wearing technique to healthy suggestions for transitioning your baby from breast milk when the time is right.

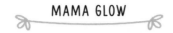

On average a pregnant woman loses 13.5 pounds within an hour of delivery. Hallelujah! You can lighten the load, girlfriend. Immediately your body will begin to make subtle changes on the road to feeling like yourself again. So sit back, hydrate with filtered water or coconut water, and let's get started bonding with your new baby. It's nursing time!

The Milky Way: Breastfeeding Support

What a miracle: not only are you powerful enough to grow and give birth to a baby, but your body can feed her, too! Although the first few days might seem rough, as you get used to the changes in your body, breastfeeding does indeed get easier and more enjoyable. I had a very positive breastfeeding experience that resulted in a robust, healthy, well-adjusted baby boy. Thankfully my mom came and helped out a lot. The first few days were challenging because I didn't know if I was doing it properly.

Weapons of Mass Production

The day my milk came in was a day I'll never forget. I gave birth on July 13, and had a successful latching for the first day and a half. On the second day, I felt my breasts become hot, painful, rock hard, and flooded with milk. They were so full that I had to buy new nursing bras that same day. I went to take a walk around the block and noticed everyone staring at my new glamorous I-put-Pamela-Anderson-to-shame breasts. Going from an A-cup to an overflowing C-borderline-D-cup was a dramatic shift for me! I had to learn how to accommodate my new breast friends.

While evidence shows that breastfeeding is the best for our babies, there is not a lot of support for breastfeeding in Western culture. The World Health Organization recommends exclusive breastfeeding for the first six months of life and that children continue to be breastfed for at least two years. Two years may sound like a long time to share your breasts, but think about the developmental and emotional benefits your child will experience from connecting to you in that way!

Breast milk is the perfect nourishment for a growing baby. It protects the baby against illness such as ear infections and the flu, and lowers the risk for asthma, diabetes, obesity, and leukemia later in life. Breastfed infants are more likely to try a wide variety of foods when they start solid baby foods and, later, table food. Breastfeeding also gives you and your baby a special connection; the majority of mothers report that breastfeeding makes them feel closer to their baby. They notice their baby becomes calmer and more satiated when at the breast. Moms tend to find it very relaxing, too.

Besides the wonderful connection you establish with your baby, breastfeeding also encourages the uterus to contract back to its normal size and helps you to drop that baby weight. It happens almost effortlessly, because you're producing milk, which uses up lots of calories. Breastfeeding can burn up to 600 calories daily. Just from breastfeeding alone you can lose a pound every week! Breastfeeding is also linked to lower maternal weight gain.

All of that said, there are challenges that can make it difficult and nearly impossible for some women to manage breastfeeding. These include stress and anxiety at home or work; extended separation of mother and baby at birth; difficulty latching that results in pain for the mother and frustration for both mother and baby; and low milk production. These issues usually arise because of stress, dehydration, and poor diet. Engorgement and improper latching are two of the most common hurdles to comfortable breastfeeding, and I will discuss each one at length.

Many women give up breastfeeding after the first few weeks postpartum due to pain and discomfort. If you're dedicated to breastfeeding, please hold out just a bit longer. Once you're over the initial hump, the experience becomes comfortable and pleasurable.

Let Your Love Come Down

The beauty and magic of the baby–breast connection is that just thinking about your little one can trigger what's called the "let-down" or "milk-ejection" reflex and start your milk flowing. When you breastfeed, your baby's suckling stimulates the nerves in your nipple. These nerves carry a message to your brain, and the hormone oxytocin is released. Oxytocin—the love hormone, which you already know all about—encourages closeness, bonding, tenderness, and feelings of elation. But it is also one of the main hormones involved in milk production. This oxytocin flows through your bloodstream to your breasts, where it causes tiny muscle cells around your milk glands to squeeze milk out of the glands and into the milk ducts—the let-down.

Once your let-down reflex is consistent (usually by two weeks after delivery), you may feel a pins-and-needles, or tingling, sensation in your breasts when you nurse or pump. Milk will usually drip or squirt from one breast while you are feeding on the other side. Sometimes your let-down will occur when you hear your baby cry or think about nursing your baby. A well-functioning let-down reflex helps ensure your breasts get emptied and your baby is easily getting milk. Over time, with continuous nursing, the sensation becomes more faint and the let-down happens with little to no feeling in the breasts at all.

GLA (Gamma Linolenic Acid) Oils

These oils are needed for optimal liver function. Your baby gets GLA from your breast milk. Since many infants never gained the important nutritional benefits of their mothers' milk, they've started off their lives being GLA-deficient. The standard American diet contains virtually no GLA, which is the second fatty acid in the omega-6 family. GLA is not only known for regulating blood sugar and providing important nutrients to the brain; it also exhibits immune-boosting properties.

The richest whole-food sources of GLA are mother's milk, spirulina micro-algae, and the seeds of borage, black currant, and evening primrose. Paul Pitchford, author of *Healing with Whole Foods,* recommends spirulina for people who were never breastfed, to foster the hormonal and mental development that may not have occurred because of lack of proper nutrition in infancy.

Engorgement

Engorgement is a sensation of fullness in the breasts that results from an over-production of milk. Within 72 hours after you give birth, a rush of breast milk becomes available to your baby. More blood flows to your breasts and some of the surrounding tissue swells, including the underarm region. The result is full, swollen, tender, engorged breasts. Although it's painful, engorgement is a good sign—it means you're producing milk abundantly. The pain won't last very long, usually up to 48 hours. It takes the body a few days to adjust to producing the right amount for your baby's needs. The body doesn't know whether you just birthed one baby or multiples, so it produces lots of milk until it gets a sense of how much is needed.

Here are some tips on managing the pain of engorgement.

- Cabbage leaves. This is a folk remedy. You peel back a layer or two of green cabbage and place it inside your nursing bra to cover your breast completely. You can leave them in for a minimum of 20 minutes, or you can leave them in until the cabbage completely wilts. The coolness and the sulfur in the cabbage—produced by the

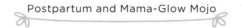

amino acid methionine—combine to act as an antibiotic and anti-irritant. This reaction in turn draws an extra flow of blood to the area, resulting in dilation of the capillaries, which is a counterirritant as well. Engorgement and inflammation are relieved, milk flows more freely, and you experience great relief.

- Take a warm shower or bath. Allow the water to gently pour directly over your breasts. The heat will cause vasodilation, meaning your milk will begin to leak in the shower, causing the breasts to deflate enough that they feel comfortable. Since the breasts aren't being stimulated, your body won't consider the leaking a feeding and you won't have to worry about producing more milk to account for the leaked milk.

- Wear comfortable clothing that doesn't cling too tightly around the chest area and doesn't cause any rubbing.

- Apply a cold compress for up to 20 minutes before a feeding. This can be helpful in reducing pain.

- Feed your baby frequently, every two to three hours at least, even if it means waking him up. This is crucial, because unrelieved engorgement can cause a permanent drop in your milk production. Try to get the first breast you use as soft and deflated as possible. If your baby is satisfied with just one breast, you can offer the other breast at the next feeding.

- While nursing, gently massage the breast to get blood flowing. This will help decrease some of the inflammation.

- Contact a lactation consultant who can show you some tips. They're usually flexible with where they see patients and can come to your home upon request. Check with your birth service provider to see if they have any partnerships with lactation consultants. (Check out the Resources section in the back of the book for more specifics.)

- A fenugreek-seed compress is a traditional remedy used in India to relieve engorgement and mastitis (inflammation of the breasts). Steep several ounces of fenugreek seeds in a cup or so of warm water. Let the seeds cool and then mash them. Place mashed seeds on a clean wet cloth while still warm, and use as a poultice on engorged or mastitic breasts to help with milk ejection and sore spots.

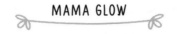
Improper Latching

Breastfeeding shouldn't be consistently painful. If you're experiencing exceptional pain while nursing, there could be an issue with the way your baby is latching onto the breast. Improper latching results in myriad problems to the new mother—including sore, cracked, and bleeding nipples, and thrush or yeast infection. If you are too sore to nurse, your milk supply will suffer and your baby won't get enough to eat. Ensuring that your baby is properly latched from day one—or correcting the problem soon thereafter—will prevent having to continually treat symptoms. Here are some tips on getting your baby properly latched, as well as treatment measures for sore, cracked nipples.

- Get started ASAP. The sooner you start breastfeeding your baby postpartum, the less likely you will experience latching challenges.

- Tease your baby. To get your baby to grasp the entire nipple and areola, you need her to open her mouth wide. You can do this by stimulating baby's rooting reflex. Try teasing your baby's lips with your nipple or finger; she should respond by opening up wide. You can also softly stroke your baby's cheek—she should automatically turn her face toward you and open wide in anticipation of feeding.

- Once your baby has her mouth open wide as if she were yawning, gently and swiftly move her head toward the breast and allow her to latch on, grasping as much of your breast into her mouth as possible.

- Position your baby correctly. Your baby's gums should be positioned on the areola, not the nipple itself. The areola is the dark circular area surrounding the nipple. Most of the areola should be covered by the baby's mouth. When properly latched, the baby initiates sucking, the milk ducts compress, and the milk is released. If your baby is instead latched on to the nipple itself, she is going to have a harder time drawing out the milk, which will frustrate her. In turn she will suck harder, which will be more painful for you.

- Malfunction? Break suction. If the baby is latched on properly you should not feel any pain. If you experience pain, or the baby is not sucking correctly, break the suction by placing your finger inside the corner of the baby's mouth near the gumline and the baby will release the breast. Reposition yourself, take a deep breath, tease the baby to open wide, and start over.

Breast milk is one of the most alkaline foods on the planet; it's a complete and perfect food. What we eat goes directly into the milk; so do our thoughts and feelings. If we're stressed out or upset, we send hormones into the bloodstream and subsequently the milk. This can upset the baby. The connection is unimaginably delicate. We must take the time to make ourselves comfortable and relax into feeding. Try to set aside a space for your feeding ritual; this is your precious bonding time with your baby. When your baby is resting make sure you get your rest, stay well hydrated, and eat foods that fortify your milk, like almonds, walnuts, chia seeds, avocado, and whole grains.

Mastitis

Mastitis is inflammation of the breasts caused by engorgement or inadequate milk removal, infrequent or skipped feedings, obstruction, or pressure on the milk duct. Sore, cracked nipples can offer a point of entry for mastitic infection, especially if there are infected cracks/fissures. If mastitis takes hold, use a cold compress on the breast between feedings to reduce inflammation. Some moms use hot compresses directly before nursing to help with the milk let-down, while others prefer to stick to the cold for pain relief.

Here are some tips to help beat mastitis.

- Nurse your baby on the mastitic breast first. Massage the breast in long strokes toward the nipple. Massage the breast often during feedings and between feedings to help open the blocked area.

- If you have a fever, take at least two to three (and, if possible, four to five) raw cloves of garlic per day. Chop a clove into small pieces, allow it to sit in open air for at least 20 minutes (the healing effects of garlic are more potent when the cut clove is exposed to oxygen), and either swallow the pieces whole like pills or add to salad dressing and eat. Raw garlic acts as a broad-spectrum antibiotic. The antimicrobial property in garlic is very sensitive to heat and is destroyed when cooked, so in order for it to heal, it needs to be raw. Note that the deodorized garlic capsules on the market are essentially useless in terms of their antimicrobial properties.

- Try a tincture. Echinacea helps stimulate the immune system and fights bacterial infections. Take one dropper full, or 20 to 25 drops,

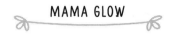
three to four times a day. Oregon grape root tincture is also a powerful antibacterial. Take one dropper full, three to four times a day.

- Vitamin C can help because it drives infection away. Try a 3000 to 5000 mg megadose every day.

- Take a very warm shower, allowing the water to gently run over your breast.

If the mastitis does not improve or gets worse after using this treatment for 24 to 48 hours, contact your doctor or midwife to see how to proceed with treatment.

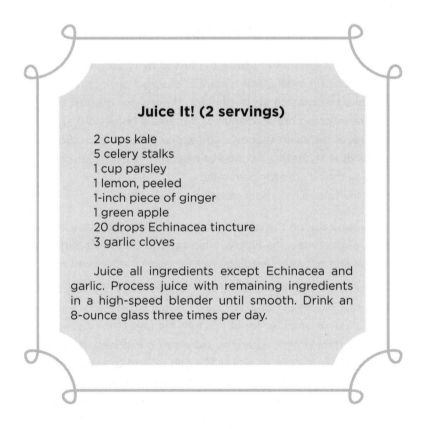

Juice It! (2 servings)

2 cups kale
5 celery stalks
1 cup parsley
1 lemon, peeled
1-inch piece of ginger
1 green apple
20 drops Echinacea tincture
3 garlic cloves

Juice all ingredients except Echinacea and garlic. Process juice with remaining ingredients in a high-speed blender until smooth. Drink an 8-ounce glass three times per day.

Thrushy Business

Another cause of great discomfort among new breastfeeding mothers is the occurrence of thrush. Thrush is an overgrowth of fungal yeast that develops on the

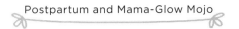

breasts because of the warm, moist environment. It passes back and forth from mother to baby during feedings, causing painful tenderness of the nipples. The result can be challenging feedings for the mother. It is important to treat thrush right away to minimize the symptoms and discomfort. Your doctor might prescribe a topical cream such as Nystatin or Lotrimin to apply to the breasts. Make sure to wash your breasts before nursing; after all, your little one will still be feeding and you don't want to pass any of these substances into the milk.

My advice is to opt for one of several natural therapies that are highly effective in treating thrush. These include:

- Gentian violet. Apply to your baby's mouth and to your affected nipple area with a cotton swab. Allow it to dry on your breast. Your baby's mouth will be purple for the three days of treatment; but it's worth it, considering the pain you will avoid in the process.

- Oil of oregano. This natural oil works on fungal, viral, and bacterial infections. Two drops under the tongue three times a day are enough (it's strong, so chase it down with water or juice). To use topically, place two drops in a teaspoon of olive oil and rub it on your baby's infected areas and your nipples.

- Yogurt. Apply plain cultured yogurt to your baby's mouth and the infected breast between feedings.

- Garlic. As discussed, its antimicrobial properties will help fight yeast overgrowth. Prepare and ingest it as described previously.

- Relax. Yeast infections are aggravated by stress, lack of rest, and poor diet. Try deep breathing, yoga, taking a solo walk, or taking a nap, and be sure to eat your glow foods!

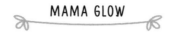

Saline Solution Boob Bath

Mix ½ teaspoon of salt in 1 cup (8 ounces) of warm water to make a saline soak. Soak the breasts in warm solution for one to two minutes after you finish feeding—long enough for the solution to get into the cracks in the nipples. Gently pat dry with a soft paper towel. Be careful not to oversoak, as too much hydration will dry out the tender skin and promote cracking. Make a fresh supply of the saline solution each day to avoid bacterial contamination. You may also buy individual-use packets of sterile saline solution if that is easier for you.

Skin-to-Skin Contact

There are now a multitude of studies that show that mothers and babies should be together, skin-to-skin, immediately after birth. The baby is happier. His temperature, heart, and breathing rates will be more stable, and his blood sugar will be more elevated. We now know that this is true not only for the baby born at term and in good health, but even for the one born prematurely. Skin-to-skin contact can contribute much to the care of the premature baby. Even babies on oxygen can be cared for skin-to-skin, and this helps reduce their need for oxygen. It keeps them more stable in other ways as well.

From the point of view of breastfeeding, babies who are kept skin-to-skin with the mother immediately after birth for at least an hour are more likely to latch on without any help. They're also more likely to latch on well, especially if the mother didn't receive medication during labor or birth. That said, I've seen C-section-born babies latch right away with no problem.

From Woe Is Me to WOW Is Me!

Have you ever had a day where you sat with your head in your hands, feeling sorry for yourself? I remember pacing back and forth, with my son in my arms, feeling helpless that he wouldn't stop crying. I, too, started to cry like a baby. Sure, we've all had those woe-is-me moments. What I want you to know is that with just a little effort, you can transform those feelings into *"wow* is me." Which is important, since your emotional energy field can transmit about 30 feet. If you are negative, people will feel that and steer clear of you. What's worse, you will attract total chaos. While you can't spiritually bypass your problems and pretend they don't exist, there are some things you *can* do. First and foremost, you can shift your attitude to one of gratitude. You can learn to love and forgive yourself, which is the Mama Glow gold standard. Once you do this, you can't stay in a funky, forlorn place for long. It just won't feel right. When you rewire yourself to seek joy, you don't have time for drama—even if it's your own.

Why am I bringing this up, you ask? Well, the time has come to talk about the baby blues. For some 80 percent of new mothers, feelings of mild to moderate depression set in a few days postpartum and can last for a few days to two weeks. The idea is not to get rid of them, but to know what you're up against. This is when you need the most support, diva. You might experience moodiness, exhaustion, and weepiness as your hormones shift and you transition from carrying your baby on the inside to caring for the baby on the outside.

More severe than the baby blues is full-blown postpartum depression, or PPD. PPD is experienced by up to 20 percent of new mothers, and can occur anytime within the first year after giving birth. Some moms feel guilt for feeling bad, and try to *should* themselves out of their feelings. That won't work, friend. Instead, you must embrace them. Let the feelings rise to the surface—then release the pain. How do you know if you have a case of the baby blues or if you're truly suffering from PPD? Here are some symptoms that may tip you off that you've got true depression on your hands:

- Irritability or hypersensitivity
- Difficulty concentrating
- Anxiety and worry
- Crying or tearfulness
- Anger
- Negative feelings such as sadness, hopelessness, helplessness, or guilt
- Loss of interest in activities you usually enjoy
- Difficulty sleeping (especially returning to sleep after waking)
- Fatigue or exhaustion
- Headaches, stomachaches, muscle or backaches

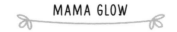

Affirmations for PPD

- I trust that this is a normal process and I welcome my feelings to the surface.

- I am grateful for this moment of emotional release.

- I am aligned with a divine power that will pull me through.

If you are in a sensitive place like this, goddess, speak with your health-care practitioner right away. You need and deserve support to help you climb out of the darkness.

Once you've talked to your practitioner, there are other things you can do on your own to get back into balance. I can't stress enough the importance of getting your hormone-regulating EFAs: flaxseed, borage, and evening primrose oils. Make sure your diet consists of primarily glow foods. Call on your support system—your partner, family, and sister circle.

Giving birth is dramatic. The transition into motherhood can be a shock for a lot of women. I encourage you to lift yourself up with affirmations when you are feeling overwhelmed and forlorn.

You are a powerful woman with the potential to create whatever you want in this life. Go ahead and grab ahold of that power—claim it as your own. How does it feel to know that you are a foxy hot mama? How does it feel to be holding your baby in your arms? You've gone through what may be the most intense experience of your life—a challenge physically, mentally, emotionally, and spiritually. The result is the birth of your beautiful baby—and your own rebirth as a fierce Mama Glow goddess. That is more WOW than anything I can imagine. Here are some tips for elevating your state of mind and mood.

- Call on your sister circle. Ask friends to come over to spend time with you.

- Get outside. Yes, it's possible that you can be in the house 24/7 and never see the light of day because you're so busy with your newborn. But getting out of the house is very important. It doesn't matter what time you get out the door, as long as you go. Have your partner or a friend stay with your baby while you bask in the sun, take a yoga class, or just go for a walk in the fresh air. The change of scenery will help you clear your head.

- Slow down. You just had a baby my dear . . . the laundry, dishes, and thank-you cards can wait. Don't do chores while your little one is asleep. That's what your squadron of sisters is for! Make sure you have someone to help you out for a little while every day.

- Be good to you. Take care of your own basic needs. Eat, drink, sleep, shower, and watch an episode of *Curb Your Enthusiasm* or whatever tickles your pickle. Make sure you have some interaction with adults who make you feel good. (Even better if they have a good sense of humor. Laughter will help ease the blues.)

- Get some rest. Not just sleeping. Try the leg drain or other restorative yoga postures you did while pregnant to relax the body as well.

- Develop a practice of giving. Being charitable and finding other small ways to be of service to those less fortunate will make you feel connected and beaming within. When you feel helpless, help someone.

- Eat mood foods. Glow foods also help you return to a place of emotional balance. All systems are connected; your emotions are largely affected by what you eat and vice versa. Some good-mood foods include foods high in B vitamins—dark leafy green veggies, brown rice, and nuts. More on mood foods follow!

Mood Foods

Serotonin is a neurotransmitter that is responsible for helping us maintain an elevated mood and stay optimistic. When serotonin levels fall, depression can be the result. Serotonin is elevated by any carbohydrate-rich food. When you need a lift, try eating carbs without protein. That way there is more tryptophan available to your brain—and tryptophan is the compound your brain converts into serotonin, making you feel good. As long as your blood sugar stays stable and your serotonin levels are high, you're in the glow zone, baby. A diet made up of mostly glow foods—all of which are serotonin boosters—along with the right amount of protein (about 3 ounces per day) will keep you feeling strong and balanced in mood.

The rise and plunge of blood sugar will determine your energy level, which in turn affects your personality and how you conduct yourself. When you feel depleted, your thoughts aren't as elevated. When you are in a hypoglycemic state (i.e., when your blood sugar is too low), kamikaze cravings arise. You'll want to eat foods that help get you through the mood—foods like coffee, bagels, and pastries.

Rice Pudding Pick-Me-Up (8 servings)

1 cup organic brown rice, short or long
   grain
1 teaspoon salt
1 tablespoon vegan butter alternative
1½ cups vanilla coconut milk (or nondairy milk of choice)
½ teaspoon pure vanilla extract
1 teaspoon cinnamon, plus more for topping
⅓ cup raw agave nectar or maple syrup,
   plus more for topping
3 tablespoons unsweetened toasted
   coconut flakes, fine (optional)

First, add the rice, 1½ cups of water, salt, and vegan butter to a medium sauce-pan. Bring to a boil over high heat. Cover with a lid, reduce heat to low, and simmer for 30 minutes, until liquid is absorbed. Next, increase heat to medium and, stir-ring constantly, add the vanilla coconut milk. Stir until liquid has been sufficiently absorbed and remove the pan from the heat. Fold in the vanilla extract, cinna-mon, and agave nectar or maple syrup. Cover with a lid and allow to sit for 10 minutes. Serve warm or store in refrigera-tor to serve cold. Sprinkle a bit of cinna-mon and a drizzle of agave nectar on top before serving. Top with toasted coconut flakes, if using.

These will give you a temporary high, followed by a slump. Many people walk through life thinking we are *supposed* to feel tired in the afternoon—and that coffee and sugar are necessary to get through the day. It's just not true! Many postpartum moms have no idea they can eat their way to a more positive outlook, but all it takes is a little information and preparation. Stock the refrigerator with complex carbohydrates and glow foods to set the mood you want.

Mood Glow Foods: Apricots, Blueberries, Broccoli, Collards, Kiwi, Peaches, Sweet potatoes, Beans, Legumes, Nuts, Avocados, Whole grains such as oatmeal and brown rice

If you want to boost your mood and have a sweet lip-smacking snack try my rice pudding recipe. It's a great dessert and kids love it, too.

Put a Sling on It! Baby-wearing

Baby-wearing is both the most popular and the most primitive way to truck around your little bundle of joy. Cultures around the world use beautiful pieces of cloth and complex wrapping techniques to secure a baby on mama's body. But what's so great about carrying your baby this way?

Besides the warmth and closeness—being able to see and feel and smell your little one up close and personal—infant carrying decreases crying by up to 50 percent and promotes infant attachment. Carried babies are happy babies. Think about it. You carry your baby for 40 weeks on the inside. She is used to the closeness! She loves being literally close to your heart. So consider carrying on with the carrying, right through the first few months of your little one's life.

But what about you? What benefits might you experience by having your baby on your body?

- Multitasking. Cook dinner, bake cookies, and soothe your baby—all at the same time. Do housework, run errands, meet up with the girls, or even check out a concert, all while providing a stimulating learning environment for your baby.

- Hands-free breastfeeding. Especially helpful while on the phone or out and about in the world.

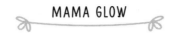

- Bonding. You're right there with your little one, learning his or her unique rhythms.

- Keeping baby close and happy. Need I elaborate?

- Getting some exercise. You can walk or hike while your baby sleeps.

- Traveling light. You can leave the stroller or carrying seat at home.

Benefits for babes:

- Less crying. Research has shown that babies who are carried cry 43 percent less overall and 54 percent less during the evening hours. In cultures where babies are carried continuously, babies cry significantly less than those in noncarrying cultures. That's something to think about!

- Mental development. Babies spend more time in a "quiet, alert state" when carried—the optimal state for learning. Their senses are stimulated, but they can also tuck away and sleep whenever they want. When carried, your baby sees the world the same way you do—instead of pondering the ceiling fan while in the crib or people's knobby knees while in the stroller. This extra stimulation promotes brain development.

- Emotional development. Babies quickly develop a sense of security and trust when they are carried. They are more likely to be securely attached to their caregivers and to explore independence at an earlier age.

- Physical and neurological development. By keeping baby close to your body's rhythms, your newborn gets in rhythm much more quickly. Your heartbeat, breathing, voice, and warmth are all familiar. Research has shown that this helps newborns, particularly premature babies, adapt to life outside the womb.

- Soothes the baby blues. Babies who are not held a lot need more verbal interaction and eye contact, just to be reassured that you're there. Carrying your baby is a great way to connect with him or her (and provide stimulation, too) without having to be engaging if you aren't feeling totally blissed out. The closeness also stimulates production of bonding hormones like oxytocin, which in elevated levels can help you shake off the baby blues.

I wore my son in a sling when he was a newborn because it allowed him to be in a dark and cozy space all tucked into himself, like when he was inside of me. I remember when his father and I got to the first pediatric visit, the nurse thought we had forgotten the baby because the sling was so close to his father's body that it looked like a fashionable scarf. (Never mind that it was in the middle of the summer!) Once he was mobile, I switched to a sling that I could wear on my back to evenly distribute the weight across both shoulders. My friends joke with me and say, "You didn't put that baby down until he was three." It sounds about right! I loved wearing my little guy in his sling. I used the sling until my son was about five so we could move through airports with ease. If I had to be in large crowds with him, it was much easier to have him on my back than in a stroller. This closeness we cultivated when Fulano was little still carries on. He has grown into a well-adjusted child who is comfortable in any situation, because he's always had support.

In the early months, practice wearing, rather than wheeling, your baby. It's a gratifying feeling to look down and see those little eyes looking back up at you. There are a ton of baby slings out there, in every color and pattern. I love the eco-friendly baby slings that Dawn Klecka of Sunshine Baby Slings handcrafts for her customers.

You're just getting acquainted with your little one, falling in love with your baby's gaze, cooing sounds, and funny faces. If breastfeeding has been a challenge, you're not alone; many women experience bumps along the road but pretty soon you will be experiencing smooth sailing. You may be wondering what foods you should be eating now that you are nursing. Well, in the next chapter, I will hook you up with boob foods for breastfeeding support.

CHAPTER 18

IN THE KITCHEN

Boob Foods

Let's explore postpartum glow foods that will support the physical and emotional changes we all encounter after birth. These foods have the added bonus of helping you return to your prebaby body. We'll talk about combining postnatal glow foods to create higher-calorie meals for moms who are nursing and on the go. We'll also talk about transitioning your baby from breastfeeding to solid food—a milestone in development for both mother and child. The Mama Glow plan offers reliable methods for ceasing milk production, as well as tasty and nutritious recipes for milk supplements and alternatives for your growing child.

Mindful eating is as important during postpartum and breastfeeding as it was during pregnancy. It helps maintain optimal health and wellness of both the growing baby and the new mother. Mother Nature designed the perfect complete nourishment for your newborn in breast milk. It is a highly alkaline, nutritive substance that contains everything your baby needs: immune factor and an impeccable balance of fats, DHA, protein, water, and happy hormones. It meets the nutritional demands and emotional needs of your baby, while promoting bonding and neurological development. At the same time, your diet during this breastfeeding period will be of the utmost importance. The dietary requirements of a nursing mom are high. Nourish yourself with the foods discussed in this chapter to support ample milk supply, adequate energy, and hormonal balance.

Your Baby's Complex Immune System

Every baby is born with passive immunity. She is protected by your immune system throughout pregnancy and leaves the womb with a supply of maternal antibodies that will keep her healthy during the first few months of life. At around six months, your baby's immune system will be able to produce its own antibodies—which is great timing, because her passively acquired antibodies will dissipate around then as well. This is one of the reasons why it is best to breastfeed exclusively for at least the first six months of life. The longer you breastfeed, the more antibodies she will obtain from you. Consider it an investment in baby's good health.

Your Milk Is the Bomb!

Breastfeeding is the best protection you can offer your little one against illness. Breast milk wards off problems more commonly found in formula-fed babies, and provides protection against allergies and gastrointestinal infections. Your milk is a good source of highly absorbable minerals, antioxidants, and other antibacterial substances that protect baby from bacterial or viral infection. Your milk is also a top-notch source of the essential fatty acids vital to proper neurological development, immune development, and growth. Not to mention that each time you breastfeed you are bonding a little more closely with your baby—getting that extra dose of oxytocin that will help you and your baby fall a little more in love. Your milk is literally a love potion.

Maintaining Your Milk Factory

While breastfeeding, you must make it a priority to look after yourself. Feeding and caring for your baby is awesome—and it's tiring, too. It helps to have lots of healthy, nutrient-packed snacks around to provide you with energy. Fruit smoothies, green juice, energy bars, yogurt, nuts, porridges, soups, hummus and crackers, sandwiches, trail mix—all help to provide sustainable energy throughout the day.

Here are some helpful tips for staying energized while breastfeeding.

- Drink enough water. I can't say this enough. Your body requires a lot more water to make breast milk, which is mostly water.

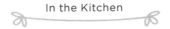

- Eat at least five portions of fruit and veggies daily. Veggies provide the fiber, vitamins, and phytonutrients needed by you and your baby. Having a fresh green juice or fruit smoothie in the morning is a great way to get an antioxidant boost to fortify your milk!

- Avoid stimulants while breastfeeding. You've heard it before. Caffeine found in coffee, tea, soda, and chocolate can cause irritability and restlessness in you and your baby, so beware. This may go without saying, but you should also limit alcohol, over-the-counter drugs, nicotine, and artificial sweeteners—all of which are bad for the baby, and bad for mama, too.

If you think your baby needs more milk, increase the number of feedings daily. The more your baby feeds, the more your breasts will produce. It's also important for you to get plenty of rest and to eat right. Try one of the many milk-making teas on the market, including Earth Mama Angel Baby's Milkmaid tea, Yogi Tea's Woman's Nursing Support, Traditional Medicinals's Organic Mother's Milk, and Tumeric's elixirs. Hot or cold, these teas are loaded with fennel, fenugreek, ginger, nettles, and more, and are designed to boost your milk production. All of these teas can be purchased online. Even if you're concerned that your milk supply is dwindling, don't start giving your baby formula or cereal. If you give formula or cereal to your baby, he or she may not want as much breast milk. This will further decrease your milk supply. It will also stretch your baby's stomach and encourage colic, eek!! Also, your baby doesn't need any solid foods before six months of age, when his iron stores start to dwindle. Which is a good reminder to continue fortifying your diet with plenty of iron even after baby is born, so he can get an extra boost through your milk.

The best diet for a breastfeeding woman is well balanced, much like your pregnancy diet but more calcium rich. Loading up on more leafy greens, wholegrain cereals and breads, beans, nuts, and seeds is key. You'll need to get enough calories—about 500 more per day than usual—and you'll need to drink more fluids to ensure adequate milk production. Talk to your doctor about taking extra calcium if you don't think you're getting enough from your diet. Medicines—even those you can buy without a prescription—can get into your milk. Don't take anything without talking to your doctor first.

If you think a food you're eating bothers your baby, stop eating it. Some will suggest avoiding strong flavors like onions, curry, and garlic while breastfeeding. I've found that generally, the dominant flavors of your diet were already in

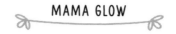
your amniotic fluid during pregnancy. Fetuses swallow a fair amount of amniotic fluid before birth, so when they taste those flavors again in their mother's breast milk, they're already accustomed to them. That said, occasionally a baby will be fussy at the breast or gassy after you eat a particular food. If you notice a pattern, avoid that food for a few days. Mothers report that babies most often object to chocolate, spices (garlic, curry, chili pepper), citrus fruits and their juices, strawberries, kiwi, pineapple, sulfur-containing veggies (onion, cabbage, garlic, cauliflower, broccoli, cucumbers, and peppers), and fruits with a laxative effect, such as cherries and prunes.

Protecting a Formula-Feeder

For a number of reasons some mamas aren't able to breastfeed exclusively. If formula milks are the only option—or if you have to supplement breast milk for any reason (surgery, medication, etc.)—then pay close attention here. First and foremost, avoid cow's milk formulas! Cow's milk is designed to take a baby calf from 65 pounds to 600 pounds within one year—that's major growth. Why would you want to feed your child a food designed to increase body mass at such an alarming rate? Instead, opt for vegetarian formulas. Also, there are milk banks for moms that would like breast milk donors. If this interests you, do a search and see if human milk is available in your area. Milkin' Mamas is a wonderful way to get human breast milk for your baby: www.milkinmamas.com.

Here are some helpful tips for formula feeding:

- Add a quarter teaspoon of infant probiotic to your baby's bottle once a day. This will provide some of the beneficial bacteria that are present in breast milk, protecting against gastrointestinal infection.

- Add a few drops of organic flaxseed oil into your baby's bottle once daily for a dose of omega-3 essential fatty acids.

- Rub the contents of a 500 mg evening primrose oil capsule onto your baby's tummy after bath time to ensure a source of omega-6s. The oil will absorb through baby's skin and into her bloodstream.

- Avoid overfeeding with the bottle. Bottle-fed babies don't have to work their jaws for the milk and often overeat. Fat cells are laid down in infancy, and an overweight baby is likely to be an overweight adult.

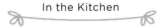

If you find your baby wants more formula than recommended, try swapping out the bottle nipple for a slower releasing one.

The Kissing Connection

So by now, you're likely to be obsessed with your baby! I know I was, I couldn't stop looking at him when he was asleep and his cheeks, feet, and belly button were the prime targets of my kisses. We've already talked about a variety of health benefits associated with breastfeeding, but did you know that breastfeeding moms can protect their babies by offering antibodies that are tailor-made to the bacteria and viruses their babies come into contact with? You have a plethora of antibodies in your own body that have been created throughout your life to protect you against certain diseases, many of which are totally irrelevant to your newborn. But others will give your baby's immune system a vital boost. When you kiss your baby's cheek, you are effectively sampling the bacteria and viruses on his face. The bacteria transfer to your body, where your immune system is stimulated to create specific antibodies to fight these pathogens. You then pass the tailor-made antibodies back to your baby through your breast milk. Each time the baby is at the breast he is getting inoculated. So keep kissing and nuzzling your baby. What a perfect miracle!

> **Glow Tip:** *Breast milk is Mother Nature's vaccine!*

Boob Foods

Boob foods are nutrient-dense, energy-packed foods that are the building blocks of your breast milk. They are glow foods that you pass through your milk to your baby. These foods help boost energy levels, too! They include the following:

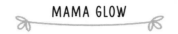

Gluten-Free Whole Grains

After yet another sleepless night, one of the best foods to boost energy for new moms in the morning is a healthy breakfast of whole-grain, gluten-free cereal. Whip up a healthy hot breakfast by stirring blueberries and almond milk into a delicious serving of oatmeal or Quinoa Porridge (Page 263), or top a smoothie with some yummy Rockstar Granola.

ROCKSTAR GRANOLA *(20 servings)*

3 ½ cups rolled oats

½ cup toasted mixed nuts

½ cup coconut flakes

¼ cup sunflower or pumpkin seeds

3 tablespoons flaxseeds

3 tablespoons sesame seeds

2 teaspoons cinnamon

¼ cup grapeseed oil

¼ cup raw agave nectar

2 tablespoons honey

1 tablespoon pure maple syrup

2 teaspoons pure vanilla extract

1 teaspoon sea salt

Preheat the oven to 375 degrees. Line a rimmed baking sheet with aluminum foil. In a large bowl, combine all ingredients, and stir well to incorporate.

Spread the mixture in an even layer on the prepared baking sheet. Bake for 20 to 30 minutes (depending on the depth of goldenness you're looking for), stirring every 10 minutes. Remove from the oven and let cool completely. Store in an airtight container for up to four weeks.

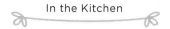

Seeds

Chia seeds, sesame seeds, sunflower seeds, pumpkin seeds—all are great for snacks. They contain zinc, iron, protein, and essential fatty acids. Throw them into a trail mix, over a salad, or into a smoothie for a protein-packed punch!

Leafy Greens

You're already well informed about the benefits of eating leafy green vegetables—including spinach, Swiss chard, and collards. Well, they're good for your baby, too. They're filled with vitamin A, which your baby needs to get from your breast milk. They're a nondairy source of dietary calcium. They've got vitamin C and iron. On top of that, green veggies are filled with heart-healthy antioxidants, and they're tasty to boot.

Algaes

Chlorella—which I like to call "bella chlorella"—is a 2.5-billion-year-old organism. It sparks immunity, greatly reduces toxins and pesticides in your system, and like all things green, comes loaded with omega-3s. Blend it up in a smoothie for green goodness. If you want something equally as versatile try the 3-billion-year-old spirulina species. Containing GLA fatty acids, more iron than beef, and more protein than soy, spirulina is super easy to digest and makes great breast milk! Finally, you can shake things up by including some wild blue-green algae. It sparks neurotransmitters, counteracts depression, and contains as many minerals as seaweed.

Fruits

Avocado: This fruit contains healthy fat and is easy to eat in a pinch—either on its own or over a salad.

Berries: Breastfeeding moms should be sure to get two or more servings of fruit or juice each day. Antioxidant-rich blueberries are an excellent choice to help you meet your quota. These satisfying and yummy berries are filled with good-for-you

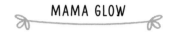

vitamins and minerals and will give you a healthy dose of carbohydrates to keep your energy levels high.

Brown Rice: If you're attempting to lose the baby weight, you might be tempted to drastically cut back on your carbohydrate consumption. But losing weight too quickly may cause you to produce less milk for the baby and leave you feeling lethargic and sluggish. It's better to incorporate healthy, whole-grain carbs like brown rice in your diet to keep your energy levels up. Nutritious, calorie-dense foods like brown rice provide your body with the nourishment it needs to produce the best quality milk for your baby.

Legumes: Beans, especially dark-colored ones like black beans and kidney beans, are a great breastfeeding food, especially for vegetarians. Not only are they rich in iron, they're a budget-friendly source of high-quality, nonanimal protein.

Suggested Meals for Breastfeeding Mamas

Here are some basic dietary suggestions for nursing mamas. I had one of my moms increase her milk production and eliminate her formula supplementation following my dietary suggestions. She also began to lose weight, after having reached a plateau for some months. I ate this way with my son and was well under my prepregnancy weight six weeks postpartum. Your diet sets the tone for how your baby will eat so choose wisely. Your little one will be joining you at the dinner table before you know it.

Breakfasts

This very important meal sets the tone for your day. It should be protein-rich and not too sweet. Morning is a great time to do something light, like a smoothie—and then have a solid meal an hour or two later. Baby will be breastfeeding around the clock, so an adequate breakfast is important for establishing rhythm and routine, as well as for self-care.

All the smoothies I share in this book are great options—but try making your own as well! Other breakfast ideas include dairy-free yogurt with berries and granola, oatmeal with berries and almond milk, tofu scramble with minced spinach, brown rice cereal, or green juice.

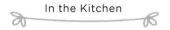
Lunches

Around midday you should be ready for a larger meal. Lunch is a great time to eat heavier foods that will take time to digest, as well as foods that will fortify your milk. Protein, fats, and complex carbohydrates are key here. Always have a side of greens with whatever you eat to help keep the bowels regular—lots of new moms suffer from constipation, so if this is a problem of yours know that you're not alone.

Salads are great options! Think quinoa and black bean salad; sandwiches; mixed greens with nuts, seeds, and some protein (whatever you like to top your salad with); hearty lentil soup; sautéed veggies and brown rice; couscous and hummus; or a veggie and brown rice burrito.

Dinners

Dinnertime should be a simple but hearty option. It should also be something that induces relaxation, so you can be prepared for the waking sleep cycles and feedings of your newborn. Any foods high in the amino acid tryptophan will promote relaxation and healthy sleep patterning, including spinach, watercress, sunflower seeds, and seaweed. All-in-one meals are great, including casseroles and stews.

Try these dinner suggestions: ratatouille; soup and salad combo; steamed squash; stewed beans; steamed veggies with brown rice and avocado, tempeh, beets, and quinoa tabbouleh.

Snacks

Snacks should be easy bites that you can prepare within minutes. You should always have a mobile pantry and snacks to take with you on the go as well. Try apple slices with almond butter, a handful of nuts, hummus and veggie slices, natural applesauce, seasoned olives and warm focaccia, chia pudding, or smoothies.

The Dry Spell: Weaning

If the time has come for you to reclaim your breasts, then it's time to take a look at a few simple recipes that can take the torture out of weaning—and make it a smoother transition for your little one. I found that my toddler was so intent on breastfeeding that I had to come up with a substitution for milk—fast! My son still drinks some of these milk alternatives. Not only are they super tasty, they're fortifying as well.

- Brazil nut milk has a similar constitution to breast milk. See recipe below.

- Coconut milk is almost identical to our own blood plasma. The jellylike coconut flesh is fatty and has a naturally sweet taste.

- Hemp milk is full of EFAs. Nutty and rich, this milk helps tremendously with brain development.

There are quite a few nut milks on the market. One of my favorite brands is Living Harvest, which recently introduced hemp milk in three flavors. You can try what's out there and also try making your own. See what your child prefers. I weaned my son on the following recipe.

BRAZIL NUT MILK *(6 servings)*

1 1/2 cups raw Brazil nuts

7 cups filtered water

Pinch of sea salt

3 dates

1 to 2 tablespoons chia seeds (optional)

Soak Brazil nuts in a bowl with 4 cups of water for one hour. Rinse. Process nuts, 3 cups of water, sea salt, and dates in a high-speed blender; strain through a fine sieve if necessary to get a thinner solution.

Want to give it a boost? Throw 1 to 2 tablespoons of chia seeds into the milk once it has been strained for a protein and fiber boost for your baby.

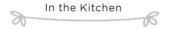

Taking Care of You

There are many foods you can eat that will help dry up your milk supply and stop production. They include sage, parsley, oregano, thyme, sorrel, and peppermint. Try making them into a tea, either individually or in mixtures. If you'd rather eat your herbs, try this Sassy Sage Pesto sauce recipe. It's a great-tasting twist on traditional pesto.

SASSY SAGE PESTO *(6 servings)*

1 cup olive oil

1 cup fresh chopped basil

3 tablespoons chopped leek

1 tablespoon fresh chopped sage

1 tablespoon chopped parsley leaves

1 cup pine nuts

1 cup olive oil

2 cloves garlic

1 teaspoon sea salt

In a food processor, gently pulse $\frac{1}{2}$ cup olive oil and remaining ingredients until finely minced. When pulsing is complete and you have a fine textured consistency, transfer into a bowl and stir in the remaining olive oil for a wonderful pesto variation.

Add this peppy pesto to a batch of your favorite pasta. Use it as a spread for sandwiches or as a topping for steamed vegetables or crudités. Or, add a dollop to the Butternut Squash Apple Soup recipe found in Appendix B.

Now that the baby is here, finding time to cook can be a challenge. Get your sister circle on the job, and have friends and family rotate with cooking duty. Preparing a shopping list while your baby is asleep and using an online grocery delivery service saves energy and time. Once you get on track with regular meals and you're at least six weeks postpartum, it's a good time to start reintegrating your yoga practice. In Chapter 19 I break down some postnatal yoga techniques that help you regain your core strength, lean out, and get you back to your prebaby body.

ON THE MAT

Claiming Your New Body

After the baby's arrival, your body will feel exhausted. And it should—labor is like running a marathon to the summit of a mountain. While you recover, there are small exercises that you can do to get things back in working order. But don't force any major exercise within the first six weeks of delivery. If you push yourself too much you will experience bleeding, which is a sign to slow down, woman. There's no rush to get back to normal. Once you accept that time works differently when you have a newborn and learn to manage your time and incorporate exercise into your day wherever it fits, you will be better off.

Micro-pelvic tilts right after delivery are a great way to reintegrate your muscles. Elevator Pelvic Pumps, or your glorified Kegels, will be helpful once your swelling subsides and you can feel the pelvic floor again. A woman's uterus expands to 500 times its normal size during pregnancy. (And a man is proud of a simple erection!) This expansion took 40 weeks, and it will take some time for your uterus to return to its previous size. The more you can rest and nurse your baby, the more your uterus will contract and tighten back up.

Move Your Body, Girl!

Once you hit the six-week benchmark, you can get back in gear and start exercising. One of the easiest ways to get moving again is on your mat. You can be with your baby and you don't have to leave your house.

Dance and Movement

I began dancing early. When I was growing up my mom would blast a Stevie Wonder or Prince record on Saturday mornings, and I would dance my heart out. She'd vacuum the floors or do the laundry, and all the while, we would dance! You don't need instructions for this one. Turn on some Jay-Z, Rihanna, Black-Eyed Peas, or Katy Perry and rock out. Whatever moves you. I mean that literally! When my son was a baby I would play the music that made me happy inside, house music or hip hop, and clean the house while swaying my hips and dancing up a sweat. This is an easy, fun, affordable way to get those lean mean curves.

Yoga and Functional Training

Get on your mat and get back into your practice. Do a gentle practice, or work yourself harder to meet the needs of your new body and lifestyle. The body weight training you get in yoga helps to protect the joints, build surrounding muscles, and rehabilitate the core—which was on vacation for nine months. Try the postures that follow to rebuild your strength postbaby.

Lunges: This strength-training exercise works the quadriceps, hamstrings, ankles, calves, and groin. If you engage your core muscles it also promotes core training, improves balance, and is excellent for improving posture. If your knees are feeling weak, you'll want to pass on this one.

How to do it: With your feet parallel at the front of the mat, step the left leg back, bend the front knee, and place your hands on your hips. Slowly lower down and rise up for 10 counts. To switch sides, pivot the feet and turn to the back of your mat so the left leg is forward. Ease down and up for 10 counts. Repeat for three sets. Then turn into a straddle position with both feet facing forward in a wide-leg stance. Inhale and lift your arms; exhale and bow forward. Relax your neck and head. Heel-toe your feet together, and roll up to stand.

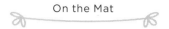

Downward-Dog Pliés: This movement combines the most basic yoga pose and the most fundamental ballet pose. It tones the inner and outer thighs, and stretches the hamstrings and calves while also working the muscles of the back and upper arms, shoulders, and wrists.

> **How to do it:** From Downward-Facing Dog, turn your heels together and let your toes turn out into a V. Squeeze your thighs together as your legs are straight and firm. On the exhale, bend your knees and squat into a frog position. Pause on the inhale, and on the next exhale straighten your legs. Do this for 10 counts. Then turn your toes forward, bend knees to the floor, and come into Child's Pose.

> **Glow Tip:** To take it up a notch, come on to the balls of the feet when the legs are straight. Try this on your second set.

Goddess Squats and Warrior Series: This powerful series for your legs, butt, abs, and arms is a stellar way to get your groove back. Refer to pages 139–140 in Chapter 11 for a description of how to do this.

Boat Pose: This pose offers a powerful abdominal workout, toning the core. It strengthens the hip flexors and spine; stimulates the kidneys, thyroid, and intestines; improves digestion; and helps relieve stress.

> **How to do it:** From a seated position on your mat bring the legs together and arms alongside your hips, and send the legs straight up to a 45-degree angle. The torso will fall back slightly, but keep your spine nice and tall. Your body will resemble a V shape. Bring your arms out straight in line with the shoulders; if it's too intense bend the knees so the shins are parallel with the floor and take both hands and grab behind the knees to help assist the lift. Here you balance on your sitz bones.

All of the postures we've visited in previous chapters work here as well. If you need restoration visit the third-trimester yoga recommendations for the restorative postures. If you'd like to follow along, visit www.mamaglow.com for the online video and let me guide you through. Getting back on track with some form of movement is important for maintaining your well-being. Our journey is coming to an end; the next and final chapter, In Your Life: You *Glow* Girl!, will prep you for spreading those wings and soaring.

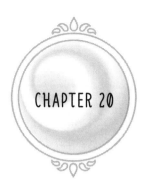

CHAPTER 20

IN YOUR LIFE

You *Glow* Girl!

When you give birth to anything—whether it be a child, a new project, a book, or a movement—you come out on the other side with something you never had before. There is a price to pay for evolution, however. You have to leave behind parts of your old self and assume the new form that comes along with transformation. Just look at the insect kingdom. A caterpillar gives up its form with total faith that it will be reborn as a butterfly. Your soul requires such a shift when you become a mother.

Radical Self-Care

Take care of yourself first, and then move on to conquering the world. When you align your body, mind, and inner diva above all else, you not only set the tone for your day, but your personal practice can help you support others. Your actions speak of how important you view yourself—how much you love and honor your relationship with self. Reignite your affirmation practice, write your new affirmations on the bathroom mirror, and place them on notecards around the house. Make time to do what you love and constantly check in with your body and spirit. I'm not just talking about getting showers in on a daily basis (which is tough in those first few weeks!). I'm talking about reclaiming your relationship with your new body and setting new boundaries so you can remain well, balanced, and lit up with glow power!

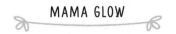

Take out your journal and answer the following questions.

- Where do I feel closed right now?
- How do I feel when I open up?
- Who are the ones in my life that light me up and make me feel more like myself?
- How does my body speak to me? What does my body say yes to, and what's a no?

Affirmations

- My body is wise and communicates when tired or inspired so that I may make the best choices for my well-being.

- I am nourishing my body and soul and I am strong.

- I accept my responsibility to speak up and take charge of my health.

Stop Multitasking, Start Uni-tasking

Women are masterful multitaskers. This skill probably evolved from ancestral times, when we were in the cave, stirring a pot with one hand and fighting off a wild animal with another, all the while balancing a happy baby on one hip. With the busy, high-speed lives we are leading these days, we are often forced to complete multiple duties at the same time. We overschedule, overcommit, overeat, and go to bed so late that we oversleep. I don't know about you, but I'm over it! I'm convinced that much of our modern stress is caused by a feeling that time is escaping us and we are racing through life just trying to get everything done. One really important lesson I learned during pregnancy and early postpartum was to slow down and do one thing at a time. I know it sounds ridiculous, but think about it. How present are you when you are doing so many things at once? You're too busy to be present at all. When, on the other hand, if you do just one thing—from start to finish—limiting your distractions, you actually get *more* done. Do the easiest things first, the things that feel pleasurable to do because you will accomplish these tasks with ease and efficiency without trying.

Uni-tasking means that rather than cooking dinner while talking on the phone, I leave my phone on the charger and prepare a meal with total concentration and awareness. Uni-tasking allows me to read a book to my son as he prepares for bed, making us both feel more relaxed as we wind down for the night. It's great that we women have the ability to juggle so many things, but when you've just had a baby, the body requires a little surrender. Slow down, listen, and reconfigure your to-do list accordingly.

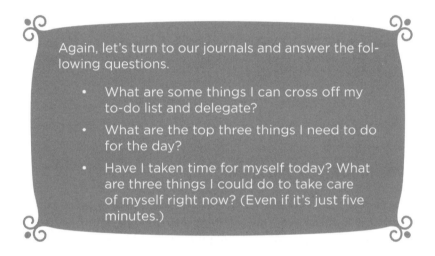

Again, let's turn to our journals and answer the following questions.

- What are some things I can cross off my to-do list and delegate?
- What are the top three things I need to do for the day?
- Have I taken time for myself today? What are three things I could do to take care of myself right now? (Even if it's just five minutes.)

The To-Be List

Move over to-do list. A to-be list is a list of words or phrases that remind us where we want to be, emotionally and spiritually. It's a gauge for how we want to be—think *calm, centered,* and *happy.* I usually start my to-be list at the beginning of the day when I wake up. Keep a mini-notebook by your bed and take a moment to write down how you want your life to feel that day. You can even post sticky notes in obvious places around your home to remind you of your list. Then, align your actions for the day with your to-be list—creating the day that you most desire, rather than getting pulled into frustration, fear, negativity, or mistrust. You can guide yourself to a balanced postpartum experience if you practice simply *being*.

Glow Tips for "Me" Time

Lyss Stern, founder of Divalysscious Moms, co-author of *If You Give a Mom a Martini: 100 Ways to Find 10 Blissful Moments for Yourself,* and fabulous mom, is a Mama Glow Icon because she knows her worth and takes at least ten minutes daily to honor herself—no matter what. Lyss actually taught me to take back my me time. Lyss offers some diva savvy tips for keeping it together once the baby arrives.

- *Start Your Day with a Royal Flush.* Drink a liter of filtered water with buffered vitamin C powder for an internal boost and walk as much as possible throughout the day.

- *Take a Bath.* Every night, no matter what, take a hot bath. Shut off that BlackBerry and light a candle, put on some calming music, and decompress from the day.

Womb Wisdom: Spark the Light!

Make time and space to reintroduce your contemplative practice. It may be different now that baby is here. Your feedings may become a perfect time to meditate with your baby in your arms. Even still, find a way to get your tail feather on a cushion and sit for a few minutes each day, to realign with the divine and remember your own divinity. To make this even more enticing, create a special place in your home where you can go to sit and look within.

To stay gorgeous, happy, and healthy in mind, body, and inner diva you have to commit to taking time for yourself and claim your space as a powerful woman. You have your own particular needs, goals, dreams, and desires and only you can design your life in a way that prioritizes them. Remember: if mama's not happy, no one is happy. My dear friend and Mama Glow Icon Heidi Krupp always says, "In order to be a great mother and great wife, you have to be great to yourself first." It's true, honey, when you take care of yourself inside and out, you can be more productive in the world. As the flight attendants in the friendly skies say, "Please secure your oxygen mask first, before assisting others."

conclusion

Glow Time!

As your glow pilot, I'm in the business of giving love and guidance, not strategic planning. I'm not against strategy; I just know what works for people. A lot of it has to do with how you feel and whether or not you accept yourself, not simply drawing up meal plans and checklists. Feelings trump methods every time. I share methodology here as a way to provide guidelines, but only you can decide the way your journey will take shape. You, my friend, are the master of your thought, the sculptor of your character, the maker of your environment, the shaper of your condition, and the co-creator of your destiny.

The universe has much bigger plans for you than you have for yourself. Explore the hidden dimensions of your life and please start doing what you love! Offer what you love, extend it beyond the boundaries of comfort and security. Be greater than yourself; that's how you grow your glow! Be the best you first, and you will be the best mama as a result. The more you harmonize with your internal nature, the healthier you will be. Wisdom is the sum of lessons learned through vital experience. Wisdom gained is the new criteria for evolution. Through this process you have become someone bigger, better, greater than you once were. You have fully stepped into your glow, full spectrum. Your shine will light the path before you and inspire those around you.

I wrote this book so I could accompany countless women across the globe as they take their unique birth journey. I wanted to give a different perspective, one that has full faith in your capabilities. I wanted you to have options that you may not have previously considered. I wanted to hold your hand as you became more confident in yourself and your power. It's been a pleasure rocking out this pregnancy! Now that you are a mother, don't ever forget that your glow is always aflame inside you, and that you can keep it ignited through self-renewal and creative discovery. Let this time be full of dreaming, bonding, growing, and glowing.

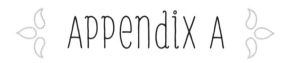

Appendix A

Quick Reference Chart of Glow Foods and Super Glow Foods

GLOW FOODS
Low and No-Starch Veggies
Arugula, asparagus, bell pepper, broccoli, Brussels sprouts, chard, chicory, collards, cucumber, garlic, green beans, kale, leek, onions, parsley, spinach, summer squash, Swiss chard, tomatoes, watercress, zucchini
Starchy Veggies
Artichoke, beans, beets, carrots, corn, peas, potatoes, pumpkin, winter squash, yams
Fruits
Apricots, bananas, blueberries, cherries, dates, figs, mangoes, pears, watermelon
Acid Fruits
Grapefruit, lemon, lime, pineapple, pomegranate
Proteins and Fats
Almonds, avocado, black beans, Brazil nuts, chickpeas, coconut oil, flaxseeds, hazelnuts, hempseed oil, lentils, mung beans, olive oil, pecans, pumpkin seeds, tempeh
Sea Vegetables
Arame, dulse, kelp, kombu, nori
Whole Grains
Amaranth, brown rice, oats, quinoa, spelt
SUPER GLOW FOODS
Acai, blue-green algae, cacao (dark chocolate), chia seeds, coconut water, goji berries, hempseeds, macá, nori, spirulina

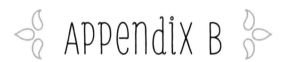

Appendix B

Mama Glow Recipes

Cooking is sacred alchemy and the more you practice the more you discover. Continue fostering your relationship with glow foods and enjoy the adventure.

The following recipes feature glow foods—powerful, nutrient-dense foods that promote optimal health and wellness, and produce the glow. The glow is a symbol of harmony within the body and mind, and an outward expression of total wellness. *Mama Glow* seeks to provide sophisticated tastes using powerful ingredients. It's all about the quality of the food that you put into your body. These ingredients, many of which are available at your neighborhood grocery store, farmers' market, or co-op, are becoming widely recognized in the mainstream market as powerful super-foods. These vegan recipes are sumptuous; they were developed during my pregnancy and postpartum experience and are by design easy to make because I know that women aren't just pregnant, they are busy, too!

SMOOTHIES AND JUICES

BASIC SMOOTHIE *(1 serving)*

10 ounces nut milk, coconut water, or apple juice

½ cup frozen fruit

½ banana, peeled

Place all ingredients in a high-speed blender and process until smooth.

PEAR PROTEIN SMOOTHIE *(4 servings)*

Vegan sources of protein come in all different forms. A seasonal pear (providing an earthy flavor) with hempseeds (providing a nutty flavor) has a rich autumn flavor. Hempseeds contain all the essential amino acids in digestible form. Pear helps regulate the bowels and cinnamon soothes the pancreas. The meal ground from the mesquite pod contains 11–17 percent protein and is high in Lysine—an important amino acid.

5 fresh pears, cored and quartered

2 cups almond milk

2 tablespoons mesquite pod meal

2 tablespoons hulled hempseeds

1 teaspoon cinnamon

2 tablespoons raw agave nectar

1 teaspoon pure vanilla extract

1 pinch sea salt

Place all ingredients in a high-speed blender and process until smooth.

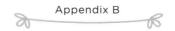

ACAI & BLUEBERRY OMEGA PROTEIN BLAST *(1 serving)*

This berry duo offers a unique blend of antioxidants and the omega fatty acids in the acai make it a complete protein. When I was pregnant and visiting Brazil, I made this smoothie every morning and my son still loves it. Acai comes in a macerated pulp in the frozen section of the grocery store. There are a handful of options out there; I use Sambazon.

1 packet acai pulp (Sambazon)

$1/2$ cup blueberries, fresh or frozen

1 $3/4$ cups apple juice or water

$1/2$ banana, peeled and sliced

1 teaspoon chia seeds

1 to 2 tablespoons Rockstar Granola (page 236) (optional)

Place first five ingredients in a high-speed blender and process until smooth. The mixture will be creamy. Place in a bowl and top with granola and the remaining half of the banana, if desired.

GOJI SUNSET SMOOTHIE *(1 serving)*

$1/2$ cup goji berries, soaked

$1/2$ banana, peeled and frozen

2 tablespoons hempseeds

2 tablespoons raw cacao powder

1 tablespoon almond butter

$1/2$ tablespoon unsweetened shredded coconut

10 ounces almond milk

Soak goji berries in water for 30 minutes. Place all ingredients in a high-speed blender and process until smooth.

ALMOND JOY SMOOTHIE *(1 serving)*

I started making this smoothie when I was doing prenatal swimming classes with Aqua Moms and needed a quick protein shake after my workout. Almonds are rich in vitamin E and help to lower blood cholesterol levels. You can use your milk of choice: rice, almond, hemp.

- 3 tablespoons almond butter
- 1 1/2 cups rice milk (or milk of choice)
- 3 pitted dates
- 1/3 banana, peeled
- 1 tablespoon raw pumpkin seeds

Place all the ingredients in a high-speed blender and process until smooth.

WILD BLUEBERRY & HEMP SHAKE *(2 servings)*

This antioxidant-rich smoothie is also loaded with easily absorbable protein. I prefer it simple with just the blueberries and hemp milk, which keeps the drink low in sugar, but it is thicker, creamier, and sweeter with the banana.

- 5 tablespoons hempseeds
- 1 1/2 cups purified water
- 3 tablespoons raw agave nectar
- 1 teaspoon pure vanilla extract
- 1 tablespoon coconut butter (optional)
- Pinch of salt
- 1 cup wild blueberries, frozen
- 1 banana, peeled and frozen (optional)

Place hempseeds, water, agave nectar, vanilla, coconut butter, and salt in a high-speed blender and process until the mixture is white, creamy, and frothy. Then add the frozen ingredients and blend again on high until smooth.

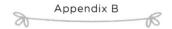

COCO-LIME SMOOTHIE *(2 servings)*

So creamy, rich, and packed with flavor, if you close your eyes you will think you are on the beach in the Caribbean.

- 1 ³/₄ cups coconut flesh
- 2 ¹/₃ cups coconut water
- 1 tablespoon fresh squeezed lime juice
- 1 ¹/₂ tablespoons raw agave nectar

Place all ingredients in a high-speed blender and process until smooth.

CACAO BREEZE SMOOTHIE *(1 serving)*

- 9 ounces Brazil nut milk or almond milk
- 3 black mission figs
- 2 pitted dates
- 2 tablespoons cacao powder
- ¹/₂ teaspoon pure vanilla extract
- Pinch of sea salt

Place all ingredients in a high-speed blender and process until smooth.

BLACKBERRY CREAM SMOOTHIE *(1 serving)*

- 4 ounces blackberries, fresh or frozen
- 1 banana, peeled
- 1 pear, cored and quartered

Place all ingredients in a high-speed blender and process until smooth.

Nut Milks

Nut milks are a highly nutritive way to experience your favorite staples without the dairy. Enjoy these with cereals, smoothies, desserts, and more.

BASIC NUT MILK RECIPE *(6 servings)*

This basic recipe is one I always like to have on hand. For chocolate milk, add 3 heaping teaspoons of organic cacao powder or carob powder, plus an additional tablespoon of agave nectar.

1 cup raw nuts

5 cups purified water

¼ cup raw agave nectar

1 tablespoon pure vanilla extract

3 teaspoons raw cacao powder (optional)

Pinch of sea salt

Soak nuts in a bowl of water completely submerged for 1 to 2 hours. Then rinse and spread across a tray lined with cloth or paper towels to air dry for an hour.

Put the nuts and water in a high-speed blender and process thoroughly on high speed. Then strain the mixture through a nut milk bag or cheesecloth and reserve the liquid. Return this liquid to the blender, add the rest of the ingredients, and blend.

INSTANT CASHEW-HEMP MILK *(3 servings)*

This is a milk I make in the mornings when running behind schedule and wanting to prepare a milk or breakfast smoothie for my son. For a sweeter cashew milk, which is how my son, Fuli, likes it, add 2 extra pitted dates.

2 ½ cups purified water

4 tablespoons cashew butter

2 tablespoons hempseeds

3 pitted dates

1 teaspoon pure vanilla extract

Pinch of sea salt

Place all ingredients in a blender and process on high until smooth and white.

APRICOT MILK *(6 servings)*

A lovely dessert milk, for those who want a hint of sweet without the guilt. Here we can use almond, cashew, or Brazil nut milk as the base. Make sure to get unsulfured dried apricots. This is a wonderful milk to use in your baby's first cereal grains.

1 cup dried apricots

2 cups purified water

5 cups milk (Brazil nut, cashew, or almond)

Pinch of sea salt

Soak dried apricots in purified water for 30 minutes. In a high-speed blender process the ingredients and blend until the texture is smooth. You can store leftovers in the refrigerator for up to four days.

GREEN JUICE *(2 servings)*

This is a juice you should have every day—before, during, and after pregnancy. You don't have to peel or deseed the fruits unless you have a preference.

- $\frac{1}{2}$ bunch celery
- 1- to 2-inch piece of ginger
- 1 lemon, peeled
- 1 cup parsley sprigs
- 4 apples, quartered
- 1 cucumber
- 2 cups curly kale
- $\frac{1}{2}$ bulb fennel (optional)

Juice all washed ingredients in a juicer.

SKIN FOOD JUICE *(2 servings)*

- 2 cups fresh pineapple chunks
- 2 apples
- 2 cucumbers
- 1-inch-thick piece of ginger
- $\frac{1}{2}$ cup fresh mint leaves

Juice all washed ingredients in a juicer.

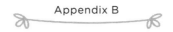

SMOOTH OPERATOR *(2 servings)*

1 large beet

2 cups fresh pineapple chunks

1 large bunch watercress

1-inch-thick piece of ginger

Juice all washed ingredients in a juicer.

//////////// BREAKFAST ////////////

QUINOA PORRIDGE *(4 servings)*

$\frac{1}{2}$ cup quinoa

$\frac{1}{4}$ teaspoon ground cinnamon

2 cups almond milk

1 teaspoon pure vanilla extract

1 tablespoon pure maple syrup

Pinch of salt

Heat a small saucepan over medium heat and add the quinoa. Add cinnamon and cook until toasted, about 3 minutes, stirring frequently. Pour in 1½ cups of the almond milk, ½ cup water, and vanilla. Then stir in the maple syrup and salt. Bring to a boil. Reduce to low heat and cook until the porridge is thick and grains are tender, about 25 minutes. Stir occasionally, especially at the end, to prevent burning. Add more water if the quinoa becomes too dry before it finishes cooking. Take ¾ of the mixture and place into a blender, whip until smooth, and return it to the saucepan with the rest of the mixture. Add the leftover almond milk, stir until even in consistency, and serve.

BREAKFAST POLENTA RECIPE *(4 servings)*

½ teaspoon salt

1 cup coarse polenta

½ cup sliced almonds, toasted

½ cup dried fruit, chopped

Honey, to taste (optional)

In a medium-sized pot, bring 4 cups of water to a boil. Add the salt and polenta. Reduce the heat and stir frequently to avoid clumping. Lower the heat and simmer for 30 to 35 minutes. If the polenta gets too thick and starts to dry out along the way, just stir in more water ¼ cup at a time.

Serve warm in bowls topped with almonds, dried fruit, and a drizzle of honey, if desired.

SNACKS

CARROT CUMIN DIP *(10 servings)*

2 pounds carrots, diced

Pinch of salt

2 teaspoons ground cumin

2 tablespoons fresh squeezed lemon juice

1 tablespoon grapeseed oil

2 tablespoons extra-virgin olive oil

Sea salt and pepper, to taste

Boil carrots in salted water until soft. Drain and allow them to cool. Place the cooked carrots, cumin, and lemon juice in a blender or food processor and blend until smooth. Drizzle in the oils and season with salt and pepper to taste.

EDAMAME SPREAD *(8 servings)*

1 pound shelled soybeans

¼ cup rice vinegar

¼ cup seasoned rice vinegar

1 ½ cups olive oil

Sea salt and pepper, to taste

In a pot of boiling water add soybeans and cook for 5 minutes until tender. Drain and allow them to cool. In a blender or food processor, pulse soybeans and vinegars until smooth. Drizzle in the oil and season with salt and pepper to taste.

BLACK-EYED PEA DIP *(8 servings)*

One 15-ounce can black-eyed peas, drained

1 pound block tofu, crushed

1 cup packed cilantro, chopped

One 4-ounce can diced green chilies

2 tablespoons grapeseed or olive oil

Sea salt and pepper, to taste

Place the first five ingredients in a food processor and process until smooth. Season with salt and pepper to taste.

LOW-FAT GUACAMOLE (8 servings)

This is one of my favorite snacks. Avocado is full of healthy fats for the glow. The peas help the guacamole to keep its color longer and add a nice sweetness to the dish.

1 cup frozen peas

3 ripe avocadoes, peeled, pitted, and crushed

Juice of 1 lime

1/4 cup packed coarsely chopped cilantro leaves

1/4 cup finely chopped red onion

Sea salt and ground black pepper, to taste

1 medium jalapeño pepper, seeded and diced (optional)

Rinse the peas in warm water, drain, and crush into a coarse paste with a fork. Add the avocado, mixing it together with the peas. Stir in the remaining ingredients and serve.

SNACK MIX (10 servings)

2 cups kamut or whole-wheat pretzels

1 cup dried carrots

1 cup spelt sesame sticks

1 cup pumpkin seeds

1 cup sunflower seeds

1/2 cup goji berries

1/2 cup raw cacao nibs

Break up the pretzels, dried carrots, and spelt sesame sticks into 1/2-inch pieces. Mix all ingredients together. Separate into 8-ounce portions and store in individual baggies.

RAW SESAME-COATED MAJOUN *(8 servings)*

This Moroccan snack is one of my favorites, a take on the classic granola bar, but so much tastier. Majoun is a tea cake that is eaten during Ramadan and is used to break the fast. I have modified it so that there is no table sugar. It's a great protein-rich snack that you can take with you on the go.

 3 cups almonds

 1 1/2 cups walnuts

 1/2 cup raw agave nectar

 1/4 teaspoon cardamom powder

 1/2 teaspoon ground ginger

 2 cups raisins

 1/4 cup sesame seeds

Using a food processor, grind the almonds and walnuts together until the mixture is fine. Place the nut mixture in a bowl and add the agave, cardamom, and ginger, mixing with a soft spatula until it becomes thick. Add in raisins and mix evenly with hands. Once thoroughly mixed, the majoun can be prepared in one of two ways. Either spread the "dough" across a cookie sheet into a thin layer, sprinkle with sesame seeds, cover with plastic wrap, and chill in the refrigerator for at least an hour. Cut into bars, then serve. Alternatively, form the dough into 8 balls and roll them in the sesame seeds. Chill in the refrigerator for one hour, then serve.

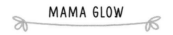
SALADS

AVOCADO, WATERCRESS & CUMIN SALAD *(4 servings)*

Avocado is amazing! Rich in monounsaturated fats, which are easily burned for energy, it helps keep the skin elastic and strong as it grows during pregnancy. It contains vitamins, A, C, and E, and more than twice the potassium of a banana.

- 2 teaspoons cumin seeds
- 1 bunch watercress, chopped
- 3 large ripe avocadoes, pitted, peeled, and thinly sliced
- 2 tablespoons Lemon Tahini Dressing (page 275)

Roast cumin seeds in a dry skillet over medium heat. Remove and crush. Place watercress on a large plate, arrange avocado on top. Sprinkle with dressing and garnish with roasted cumin.

BRAZIL NUTS WITH SUN-DRIED TOMATOES & BEAN SALAD *(4 servings)*

Brazil nuts are a great source of protein and fat. Due to their high selenium (selenium is a powerful antioxidant) content they are a complete protein, meaning they contain all the amino acids necessary for optimal growth in humans. They are also a very good source of zinc (essential to digestion and metabolism).

- 1 pound French beans, ends cut off
- 3 ounces sun-dried tomatoes, sliced
- 1 cup Brazil nuts, chopped
- 1 tablespoon olive oil
- Sea salt and pepper, to taste

Steam the beans until tender. Place the rest of the ingredients in a bowl, mix in the beans while still hot, then serve.

ROCKIN' KALE SALAD *(4 servings)*

1 bunch of curly kale

2 avocadoes, halved, peeled, pitted, and diced

3 1/2 tablespoons fresh squeezed lemon juice

2 large tomatoes

1/2 cup mung bean sprouts (optional)

1 tablespoon extra-virgin olive oil

Sea salt, to taste

Pinch of cayenne pepper

Wash the kale well. Remove the leaves from the inner stem with your hands or a knife. Place the leaves into a large mixing bowl and with your hands rip them into small bite-sized pieces. Add the diced avocado and lemon juice. Dice the tomatoes and add to the bowl. Toss in the sprouts, olive oil, sea salt, and cayenne. Serve immediately.

CARDAMOM CARROT SALAD *(6 servings)*

I love carrots, especially heirloom varieties that come in purples, reds, and yellows. This salad is a favorite in the autumn and winter because carrots are sweeter then. This is easy to make, and if you get heirloom carrots while in season, you will have a vibrant dish full of autumnal colors. Carrots contain tons of carotene, which the body converts to vitamin A. It's a versatile vegetable and an excellent source of vitamins B and C.

1 pound carrots

½ cup cilantro

3 tablespoons olive oil or vegan butter

2 teaspoons cardamom powder (or freshly ground)

1 tablespoon raw agave nectar

½ teaspoon fine sea salt

Black pepper, to taste

Wash the carrots and lightly peel. Cut in half or quarter sticks. Bring a pot of water to a boil, with just enough water to submerge the carrots. Add the carrots and cook for about 2 minutes. Remove the carrots from the hot water and place them in a large bowl of about 8 cups of ice-cold water to stop the cooking process. Once they are cool to the touch, drain the carrots and set them aside in a large bowl. Dice the cilantro finely and add to the bowl of carrots. Place the oil in a saucepan over medium heat, and then add the cardamom, agave, salt, and pepper. Cook until warm. Pour the mixture over the carrots and cilantro, mixing thoroughly until the cilantro and sauce have been evenly distributed. Serve right away or keep refrigerated for up to a week.

TOMATO & GARLIC SALAD *(6 servings)*

This raw salad is amazing in the summertime and early autumn when tomatoes are at their finest. Fresh herbs and garlic have antibacterial and antifungal properties, which boost the immune system. This is a great five-minute meal and you will savor every bite.

- 2 pounds ripe tomatoes, sliced
- 4 tablespoons fresh wild marjoram
- 2 garlic cloves, finely chopped
- 6 tablespoons olive oil
- 2 tablespoons balsamic vinegar
- Salt and pepper, to taste

Arrange the tomatoes on a plate and sprinkle with the remaining ingredients.

TUNISIAN KALE SALAD *(8 servings)*

Kale is one of the darkest leafy greens, and it packs in a heap of nutrients including calcium, iron, vitamins A and C, and chlorophyll. It tonifies the stomach, liver, and immune system. If you are a huge greens gal, you will love this salad. And if you aren't you may well still enjoy it because the dressing is so tasty!

2 ½ bunches dinosaur or lacinato kale

1 ½ cups pitted green olives

1 ½ cups diced red bell pepper

1 cup hempseeds

For the dressing:

1 cup raw tahini

½ cup lemon juice

4 tablespoons extra-virgin olive oil

4 tablespoons nama shoyu soy sauce

1 tablespoon raw agave nectar

1 ounce grated ginger

1 teaspoon spicy curry powder

1 teaspoon cayenne pepper

1 teaspoon sea salt

Slice the kale by the bunch across the ribs to get thin slices, and place in a large bowl. Add the olives, bell pepper, and hempseeds. Blend dressing ingredients to get a thick consistency, then pour over the kale and mix thoroughly. Can be served right away or made a day ahead. If you don't plan to serve immediately, wait to dress the greens so they don't get soggy.

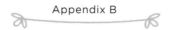

NOT YOUR GRANDMA'S COLESLAW SALAD *(4 servings)*

1 tablespoon chopped scallion

1 ½ cups carrots

½ cup purple cabbage

½ cup burdock (optional)

For the dressing:

2 large pitted dates

2 tablespoons chopped tomato

¼ cup lemon juice

¼ cup nama shoyu soy sauce

1-inch thick piece ginger, chopped

¼ teaspoon chopped garlic

½ teaspoon sesame oil

¼ teaspoon chopped jalapeño

Pinch of white or black pepper

Julienne the veggies and put them in a large bowl. Place ingredients for the dressing in a food processor or blender and mix. It should be a saucy consistency. Pour the dressing over the salad and toss.

DRESSINGS

SUN-DRIED TOMATO VINAIGRETTE *(10 servings)*

1/2 cup olive oil

1/2 cup raw apple cider vinegar

1/2 cup nama shoyu soy sauce

1/2 cup sun-dried tomatoes

1/4 cup fresh squeezed lemon juice

3 garlic cloves, peeled

Process all ingredients in a high-speed blender until smooth.

RICH GARLIC DRESSING *(4 servings)*

4 tablespoons balsamic vinegar

1 tablespoon pure maple syrup

1 tablespoon Dijon mustard

2 garlic cloves, crushed

1/2 cup olive oil

Sea salt and freshly ground pepper, to taste

In a bowl, whisk together the first four ingredients. Then add the oil very slowly, whisking continuously until the dressing starts to emulsify. Season with salt and pepper.

LEMON TAHINI DRESSING *(6 servings)*

2 tablespoons fresh squeezed lemon juice

1 tablespoon tahini

1 tablespoon pure maple syrup

1 tablespoon Dijon mustard

7 tablespoons olive oil

Sea salt and freshly ground pepper, to taste

In a bowl, whisk together all ingredients until the dressing has a thick, smooth consistency.

LUSCIOUS DILL DRESSING *(4 servings)*

1 cup Thai coconut water, fresh or bottled

1 cup raw macadamia nuts, pine nuts, or cashews

$\frac{1}{3}$ cup fresh squeezed lemon juice

1 bunch fresh dill with stems

3 garlic cloves, peeled

$\frac{1}{2}$ teaspoon sea salt

Process all ingredients in a high-speed blender until smooth.

RELISHES, SALSAS & CREAMS, OH MY!

MAMA'S MANGO-AVO-SERRANO RELISH *(10 servings)*

This is a great condiment to have on hand to accompany Latin-inspired dishes.

2 tablespoons olive oil

½ medium red onion, finely diced

¼ cup finely diced red bell pepper

¼ cup finely diced yellow bell pepper

½ cup orange juice

½ cup fresh squeezed lime juice

1 teaspoon sea salt

1 teaspoon raw agave nectar

2 mangoes, peeled and cubed

2 tablespoons minced serrano or jalapeño chili peppers

3 tablespoons chopped cilantro

½ cup diced cucumber

1 avocado (a little under-ripe), pitted, peeled, and cubed

Mix all ingredients together in a bowl, folding in the avocadoes last. Store in the refrigerator for up to five days.

LEMON-FENNEL-OLIVE RELISH *(10 servings)*

This sumptuous relish is a great spread on crackers or toasted bread.

1/4 cup olive oil

1/2 cup fresh squeezed lemon juice

1/4 cup chopped Italian parsley

1/3 cup minced red onion

1 cup diced fennel bulb

1/2 cup chopped fennel fronds

2 tablespoons lemon zest

1/2 cup chopped olives (green or kalamata)

1 teaspoon raw agave nectar

1/4 cup orange juice

1 teaspoon sherry vinegar

Mix all ingredients together in a mixing bowl and store in the refrigerator for up to a week.

SWEET BABY CORN RELISH *(10 servings)*

This is a wonderful condiment to add to your rice and beans, and it is great served over a bed of salad greens with quinoa. Or serve a dollop on top of a lentil veggie burger.

½ cup finely chopped red onion

½ cup extra-virgin olive oil

3 cups corn kernels, fresh or frozen

½ cup diced red bell pepper

½ cup diced yellow bell pepper

1 teaspoon raw agave nectar

1 teaspoon sea salt

½ cup rice vinegar

2 tablespoons chopped green onions

1 large jalapeño, seeded and minced

2 tablespoons orange juice

1 tablespoon fresh squeezed lemon juice

Place red onion, olive oil, corn, bell peppers, agave, salt, and vinegar in a saucepan and cook over medium heat for 7 to 10 minutes. Then fold in green onions and jalapeño. Add the orange and lemon juices and stir for 2 minutes. Remove from heat and cool. Can be stored in the refrigerator for up to five days.

PICO DE GALLO *(6 servings)*

1 cup fresh diced tomato, with seeds removed

¼ cup minced red onion

¼ cup chopped cilantro

2 tablespoons fresh squeezed lime juice

½ teaspoon sea salt

Mix all ingredients together in a bowl. Salt to taste. Can be stored in the refrigerator for up to five days.

PINEAPPLE-MANGO SALSA *(8 servings)*

$1/2$ cup finely diced pineapple

$1/2$ cup finely diced mango

$1/4$ cup finely diced red pepper

1 tablespoon minced jalapeño

1 tablespoon chopped cilantro

2 teaspoons fresh squeezed lime juice

$1/4$ teaspoon sea salt

Fold all ingredients together in a bowl until blended evenly. Can be stored in the refrigerator for up to three days.

MACADAMIA NUT SOUR CREAM *(8 servings)*

This is healthier and much tastier than the dairy version. It takes just a few minutes to prepare.

1 cup macadamia nuts

$1/4$ cup olive oil

1 tablespoon fresh squeezed lemon juice

$1/2$ teaspoon sea salt

Soak macadamia nuts for 2 hours. Rinse and spread across a tray lined with cloth or paper towels to air dry for an hour.

Place all ingredients and $1/2$ cup water in high-speed blender and process until smooth. Will keep in the refrigerator for five to six days.

/////////////// SOUPS ///////////////

SPICY CHICKPEA & LENTIL SOUP *(10 servings)*

This soup is said to have warmed the Berbers during the cold winters in the Atlas Mountains. The spices and tomatoes modernize this dish. Serve with a small side of brown rice to keep yourself toasty during the winter. The chickpeas and fava beans should be soaked overnight. If you don't have time to soak and boil the beans, you may use canned chickpeas and frozen fava beans. This is one of my favorite dishes, and my son loves it, too.

1 heaping cup dried chickpeas

1 heaping cup dried fava beans

3 tablespoons olive oil

2 onions, sliced

½ teaspoon ground ginger

½ teaspoon ground turmeric

1 teaspoon ground cinnamon

Pinch of saffron threads

Two 14-ounce cans chopped tomatoes

2 teaspoons raw agave nectar

¾ cup brown or green lentils, rinsed

7 ½ cups vegetable stock or water

½ cup chopped cilantro

½ cup chopped Italian parsley

Sea salt and freshly ground pepper, to taste

Soak the chickpeas and fava beans overnight in a bowl with 8 cups of water, or in separate bowls in 4 cups of water each. Boil beans together until tender, for approximately 30 minutes. Set aside. Heat the olive oil in a large pan, add the onions and stir over low heat for 15 minutes or until soft and translucent. Add the ginger, turmeric, cinnamon, and saffron, then tomatoes and agave. Stir in the lentils and pour in the stock or water. Bring the liquid to a boil, reduce the heat, cover and simmer for about 25 minutes until lentils are tender. Stir in the cooked chickpeas and fava beans, bring back to a boil, and simmer for 10 to 15 minutes. Stir in the fresh herbs and season with salt and pepper to taste. Serve piping hot.

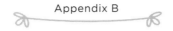
MAGIC MUSHROOM SOUP *(8 servings)*

3 tablespoons extra-virgin olive oil

1 pound assorted fresh mushrooms, cut into bite-sized pieces

Fine sea salt and freshly ground pepper, to taste

1 medium yellow onion, finely chopped

1 medium red onion, finely chopped

2 to 3 tablespoons nama shoyu soy sauce

1 $\frac{1}{2}$ cups cooked pearled barley

6 cups vegetable broth

$\frac{1}{4}$ teaspoon toasted sesame oil

1 tablespoon finely chopped chives

In a 5-quart soup pot or Dutch oven, heat 2 tablespoons of olive oil over medium-high heat. Stir in the mushrooms and season with salt and pepper. Cook for about 8 minutes, stirring a couple times along the way, until the mushrooms release their liquid and they are deeply browned. Remove the mushrooms from the pan, and set them aside on a plate.

Using the same pot, heat the remaining tablespoon of oil over medium-high heat. Stir in the onions and cook for a few minutes until tender. Stir in 2 tablespoons of the soy sauce, the barley, and then the vegetable broth. Bring to a boil, and then reduce the heat to a simmer. Add the mushrooms and cook another 10 minutes or so. Stir in the toasted sesame oil and taste. You might want to add the remaining tablespoon of soy sauce, particularly if your broth isn't very salty. And you might want to add more toasted sesame oil a few drops at a time. Serve sprinkled with chives.

CARROT AVOCADO SUN SOUP *(4 servings)*

1 large avocado

2 cups carrot juice

1 tablespoon minced ginger

1 $\frac{1}{2}$ tablespoons fresh squeezed lemon juice

$\frac{1}{2}$ jalapeño pepper, seeded

$\frac{1}{2}$ teaspoon chopped garlic

$\frac{1}{4}$ teaspoon cayenne pepper

15 large basil leaves

1 $\frac{1}{2}$ tablespoons olive oil

4 fresh mint leaves

Peel and pit avocado. Cut avocado in half, slicing one half into 4 slices. Dice remaining half and place in high-speed blender with other ingredients, except mint. Puree until smooth. Pour into four bowls and garnish with mint and avocado slices.

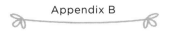

RAW HEARTY CHUNKY CHILI *(8 servings)*

I've adapted this traditional favorite into a raw recipe. This chili doesn't have beans but has portobello mushrooms as the main ingredient. It takes just a few minutes to make, and it's a great snack. Feel free to experiment with the ingredients, like swapping walnuts for the almonds. When I was pregnant this was one of my go-to meals during the cooler months—the spices made me feel warm and cozy.

1 cup almonds

1 portobello mushroom, finely chopped

½ cup minced celery

½ cup chopped red onion

½ cup chopped green bell pepper

1 cup chopped carrots

1 ½ cups sun-dried tomatoes

1 clove garlic, peeled

¼ cup nama shoyu soy sauce

1 tablespoon raw apple cider vinegar

1 tablespoon olive oil

1 tablespoon raw agave nectar

1 tablespoon cumin

1 tablespoon dry oregano

2 teaspoons fresh oregano

2 teaspoons chili powder

¼ teaspoon cayenne pepper

Soak almonds for a minimum of 3 hours and up to 8 hours. Then rinse and spread across a tray lined with cloth or paper towels to air dry for an hour.

Place mushrooms, celery, onions, and green bell pepper in a large bowl. Pulse almonds and carrots in a food processor until they reach a chunky consistency. Then add to bowl. Blend remaining ingredients and 2 cups of water in high-speed blender until smooth. Pour into bowl and mix all together until well combined. Store in the refrigerator for up to four days. Remove from the refrigerator 30 minutes or so before eating.

BUTTERNUT SQUASH APPLE SOUP *(6 servings)*

2 tablespoons olive oil

1 small onion, chopped

1 stalk celery, chopped

1 medium carrot, chopped

1 large apple, peeled, cored, and chopped

2 medium potatoes, peeled and cubed

1 medium butternut squash, peeled, seeded, and cubed

One 32-ounce container vegetable stock

Sea salt and freshly ground black pepper, to taste

In a large pot heat the olive oil on medium heat, and sauté the onion, celery, carrot, apple, potatoes, and squash for 5 minutes, or until lightly browned. Pour in enough of the vegetable stock to cover vegetables. Bring to a boil. Reduce heat to low, cover the pot, and simmer for 40 minutes, or until all vegetables are tender. Transfer the soup to a blender, and blend until smooth. Return to the pot, and mix in any remaining stock to attain desired consistency. Season with salt and pepper.

GAZPACHO *(6 servings)*

2 to 3 pounds ripe tomatoes, roughly chopped

4 to 6 garlic cloves, peeled

1 large cucumber, peeled, seeded, and roughly chopped

1 mild green chili pepper, seeded and roughly chopped

1 red bell pepper, cored, seeded, and roughly chopped

1 small yellow onion, roughly chopped

$\frac{1}{3}$ to $\frac{1}{2}$ cup extra-virgin olive oil

Sea salt, to taste

Put tomatoes, garlic, cucumbers, chili pepper, red bell pepper, and onions into a large bowl and toss to combine. Working in batches, puree vegetables in a blender or food processor until smooth, adding $\frac{1}{4}$ cup water if mixture seems too thick. Strain puree through a medium sieve, discarding peels and seeds.

Place half of the strained puree back into the food processor, and puree again. With the food processor still running, drizzle in the oil. Return to the bowl with remaining puree; stir well and season with salt. Cover and chill thoroughly, then ladle into bowls and serve.

SAVORY SIDES

CRANBERRY BALSAMIC BRUSSELS SPROUTS *(8 servings)*

This is a great dish for the holidays.

> 1/4 cup safflower oil
>
> One 16-ounce bag of fresh Brussels sprouts, preferably organic
>
> 2 1/2 tablespoons balsamic vinegar
>
> 1/2 cup dried cranberries
>
> 1/4 teaspoon black pepper
>
> 1/2 cup chopped raw pecans (optional)
>
> Sea salt, to taste

Add oil to a hot skillet over high heat. Add sprouts, 2 tablespoons of balsamic vinegar, and 2 tablespoons of water. Cover with a lid and allow sprouts to steam cook for 2 to 4 minutes or until they become tender. Remove the lid and add the remaining 1/2 tablespoon of balsamic vinegar. Sauté for another 3 to 4 minutes, adding more water if needed. Remove from the heat, and add the dried cranberries, pepper, and pecans, if using. Season with salt as needed.

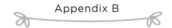

CRANBERRY-CURRY COUSCOUS IN A HURRY *(8 servings)*

This is a great dish to accompany the Vegan Moroccan Tagine found on page 296.

2 cups vegetable stock

2 cups couscous

1 teaspoon curry powder

1 teaspoon finely diced preserved lemon

1 shallot, finely diced

3 tablespoons extra-virgin olive oil

$\frac{1}{2}$ cup dried cranberries

Sea salt and freshly ground pepper, to taste

Bring vegetable stock to a boil. Place uncooked couscous in a large bowl. Pour the boiling stock in a separate bowl and add curry powder, preserved lemon, shallot, and olive oil. Mix well. Pour the stock mixture over the couscous, add the cranberries, mix, and cover immediately. Let stand for 10 minutes. Uncover and fluff with fork. Season with salt and pepper.

SPROUTED TABBOULEH *(8 servings)*

I love this side dish because bulgur is such a hearty grain, yet it's easy to manipulate. This sprouted tabbouleh doesn't require you to cook anything—simply soaking the grain allows it to bloom open. If it soaks overnight it will be fully sprouted, increasing its nutritional profile. It's nice and fluffy and easily digested.

1 cup bulgur

5 cups filtered water

1/2 cup olive oil

1/2 cup fresh squeezed lemon juice

1 teaspoon sea salt

1/4 teaspoon cayenne pepper

2 cups diced tomato (2 large diced, seeded)

2 cups chopped parsley

1 cup chopped cilantro

1/2 cup finely chopped mint leaves

1/2 cup chopped onion

1/2 cup chopped scallion

1/2 teaspoon ground allspice

Soak the bulgur in filtered water for at least 2 hours. Rinse and drain the bulgur; it will have swollen to approximately double the size. Spread onto an absorbent paper towel and allow it to dry completely for an hour then return it to a mixing bowl. Add the oil, lemon juice, salt, and cayenne pepper. Allow to stand for 1 to 2 hours, if possible, to allow the flavors to develop. Stir in the remaining ingredients. Serve cool. Will keep in the refrigerator for about a week, but it's best if eaten within three to four days.

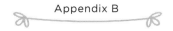

GINGERLY MASHED SWEET POTATOES WITH LIME *(4 servings)*

2 pounds sweet potatoes, peeled and cut into 1-inch cubes

2 teaspoons sea salt

1 garlic clove

1 teaspoon extra-virgin olive oil

1 tablespoon fresh peeled, grated ginger

1 tablespoon minced shallot

1 small Thai chili or jalapeño, seeded and minced (optional)

3 tablespoons vegan butter alternative

2 tablespoons pure maple syrup or raw agave nectar

1 tablespoon finely chopped cilantro

1 tablespoon fresh squeezed lime juice

Sea salt and freshly ground pepper, to taste

Place potatoes in a large saucepan, and fill it with enough cold water to cover the potatoes by 1 inch. Add the salt and garlic and bring the water to boil. Reduce the heat and simmer until tender (should be easily pierced by a paring knife), about 25 minutes. Meanwhile in a small skillet, heat the oil and add the ginger, shallot, and chili, if using. Sauté for about 2 minutes until soft and fragrant, stirring frequently. Remove from the heat and set aside.

When the potatoes and garlic are done, drain (retaining $\frac{1}{2}$ cup of water for mashing consistency) and return them to the saucepan. Add the cooked ginger mixture, vegan butter, maple syrup, cilantro, and lime juice. Mash to desired consistency. Season with sea salt and pepper to taste.

SWEET LEMONGRASS AND LIME CORN *(6 servings)*

Tired of the same old corn on the cob—boiled and lathered in butter? Well, try this corn recipe on for size. The aromatic lemongrass enhances the sweetness and chilies add some heat! This is a great side dish to almost any meal; it packs easily for lunch and can be tossed over salad.

3 tablespoons vegan butter alternative

2 tablespoons olive oil

1 to 2 stems lemongrass, bruised and cut in half

2 small Thai chilies, seeded and finely chopped (optional)

2 tablespoons fresh squeezed lime juice

2 teaspoons lime zest

1-inch-thick piece ginger, grated

Two 16-ounce bags frozen corn

1 cup diced red bell pepper

2 teaspoons finely chopped cilantro leaves

Sea salt, to taste

Heat the vegan butter and oil in a large saucepan over low heat. Add lemongrass and braise gently for 5 minutes, then remove from the pan. Add the chili and cook for 2 minutes. Stir in the lime juice, lime zest, and ginger. Add a few tablespoons of water and the corn. Cover and cook, shaking the pan frequently. Add the red bell pepper, and cook for 5 to 8 minutes until corn is tender. Stir in the cilantro. Season with a bit of sea salt and serve hot.

TUNISIAN PLANTAINS *(6 servings)*

Sweet and crisp, baked slices of plantain are a great snack. This play on one of my favorite Latin side dishes uses the potassium-rich plantains and packs them with flavors from the East. The Za'atar spice mixture is popular throughout North Africa and is also used in Turkey and Jordan. You can find it in a spice market or specialty grocery store. Find plantains at Latin and Caribbean markets or specialty markets like Whole Foods. Toast the herbs to get an aromatic effect and increase the intensity of color.

2 large green plantains

2 tablespoons coconut oil

1 dried chili, crushed

1 tablespoon Za'atar seasoning

Sea salt, to taste

Preheat the oven to 350 degrees. Peel the plantains by cutting both ends, making a long incision lengthwise and then removing the peel. Cut into $1/4$- to $1/2$-inch slices and place plantains on a well-oiled baking sheet, using the coconut oil. Put in the oven and flip the slices after about 7 minutes. When browned on both sides remove from the oven and while still warm place in a shallow bowl and sprinkle with dried chili, Za'atar seasoning, and salt. Toss thoroughly and serve.

JALAPEÑO HUMMUS *(6 servings)*

I love to make raw hummus! When I have the foresight I will soak and sprout the garbanzo beans myself, and sometimes I buy them from the store sprouted in the produce section. In a pinch you can use canned beans.

4 to 6 garlic cloves, finely minced

$\frac{1}{2}$ cup sprouted garbanzo beans

1 $\frac{1}{2}$ cups peeled and diced zucchini

2 tablespoons tahini

$\frac{1}{4}$ cup fresh squeezed lime juice

1 teaspoon sea salt

2 tablespoons ground cumin

$\frac{1}{3}$ cup olive oil

2 jalapeño peppers, seeded and minced

$\frac{1}{2}$ cup minced cilantro, plus more for garnish

Pinch of red pepper flakes

In a food processor, chop the garlic by pulsing a few times, then add the garbanzo beans, zucchini, tahini, lime juice, salt, and cumin, and puree. Slowly drizzle in the olive oil while it is pureeing. Add the minced jalapeño and cilantro and pulse for several seconds. Garnish with chopped cilantro and red pepper flakes.

GREEN CHILI CORNBREAD *(8 servings)*

This was inspired by my recent visits to Arizona, where my mother now resides. It is a unique spin on regular cornbread and pairs well with my Raw Hearty Chunky Chili (page 283) or Mexi-Cali Black Beans (page 294).

1 cup cornmeal

1 ½ cups whole-wheat flour

1 teaspoon sea salt

1 teaspoon baking soda

2 scant tablespoons baking powder

1 ½ cups coconut milk

2 cups frozen corn kernels

¼ cup coconut oil, plus more for pan

2 tablespoons pure maple syrup

1 cup hot green chilies, seeded and chopped

Preheat oven to 350 degrees. In a large mixing bowl whisk the dry ingredients together. Then add the coconut milk, corn, oil, and maple syrup, and mix thoroughly. In an oiled 9-inch pan, pour in half the batter, then cover with half the chilies. Repeat sequence with remaining batter and chilies. Bake for approximately 40 minutes. Allow to cool for at least 10 minutes prior to serving.

MEXI-CALI BLACK BEANS *(8 servings)*

These beans are a good source of protein and are especially filling. They're great for dinner or to pack for lunch on the go along with quinoa and avocado or brown rice. Serve with my Pico de Gallo (page 278) or Mama's Mango-Avo-Serrano Relish (page 276).

3 cups dried black beans

1 tablespoon olive oil

1 cup chopped onion

4 garlic cloves, minced

2 teaspoons oregano

2 teaspoons sage

2 teaspoons thyme

3 teaspoons cumin

1 teaspoon ancho powder

1 teaspoon chipotle powder

2 dried bay leaves

2 tablespoons kosher salt

½ cup chopped green onion

Soak beans in 8 cups of water overnight. Sort out withered, discolored, or abnormal beans. Rinse and drain the beans; discard the water. Heat the oil in a 5-quart saucepan and add the onions and garlic. Cook on medium heat for 5 minutes. Toast the herbs, cumin, ancho powder, and chipotle powder in a small skillet until fragrant, then add this to the onion-garlic mixture. Add the black beans and bay leaves along with enough water to cover by 3 inches. Cover and cook over medium heat until beans begin to soften, about 1 hour. Add kosher salt and stir. Continue to cook gently until fully tender for another hour. Split into eight portions and sprinkle a teaspoon of chopped green onion on top of each when serving.

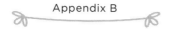

COCONUT CHAPATIS *(9 servings)*

A lovely pan-fried bread with the rich flavor of coconut. Perfect eaten alone or used as a wrap. A great alternative to pita bread. If you are avoiding gluten, you can substitute wheat flour with garbanzo flour.

- 4 cups wheat flour (or garbanzo flour)
- 1/2 teaspoon sea salt
- 1 1/4 cups coconut milk
- 1 tablespoon coconut oil

Place flour and salt in a large bowl and slowly stir in coconut milk. Mix the dough and form into a ball with your hands. Knead it on a floured surface until the dough becomes firm and pliable. Dust with more flour if the dough is too sticky. Divide into nine equal-sized balls; roll out each to about 6 inches in diameter and let them stand for 15 minutes. Brush a heavy frying pan with coconut oil and cook chapatis on each side for 3 to 4 minutes until golden brown. Serve hot!

ENTRÉES

VEGAN MOROCCAN TAGINE *(6 servings)*

Tagine is a traditional stew that is named after the conical-shaped earthenware vessel in which it is cooked, but you can also prepare it in a Dutch oven. My Bedouin friends showed me how to prepare this dish without animal products. Serve with couscous and transport yourself to the Kasbah without ever leaving home.

   3 tablespoons extra-virgin olive oil

   3 tablespoons vegan butter alternative or coconut oil

   Two 8-ounce packages tempeh, cut into 1/2-inch chunks

   1 tablespoon ground ginger

   2 teaspoons ground turmeric

   1 teaspoon ground allspice

   1 tablespoon smoked paprika

   1/8 teaspoon saffron threads

   1 large onion, diced

   2 tablespoons minced garlic

   3 cups vegetable stock

   2 tablespoons finely diced preserved lemon

   1 cup pitted black kalamata olives

   Sea salt and freshly ground pepper, to taste

   1/2 teaspoon chopped cilantro, for garnish

In a large Dutch oven heat oil and vegan butter or coconut oil over high heat. Add the tempeh and lightly brown it on each side, about 1 1/2 minutes per side. Transfer to a plate. Reduce the heat to medium-low.

Add the ginger, turmeric, allspice, paprika, and saffron, and cook for 30 seconds, stirring constantly. Add the onion and garlic, and cook for 3 minutes or until onion turns transparent.

Return the tempeh to the skillet, add the stock and preserved lemon, and stir well. Cover and cook over medium heat for about 10 minutes. Remove from heat and

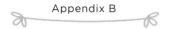

add olives. Season with salt and pepper, stir, and prepare to serve with couscous. Sprinkle a generous amount of cilantro on top.

COLLARD WRAPS WITH TAMARIND ORANGE SAUCE *(8 servings)*

These mini wraps are a great way to bulk up on fiber from greens while enjoying the sweet fruity taste of mango and orange.

For the wraps:

  ¼ cup raw agave nectar

  ½ cup fresh squeezed lemon juice

  2 tablespoons chopped ginger

  1 tablespoon nama shoyu soy sauce

  1 cup almond butter

  ½ head cabbage, shredded

  ⅔ cup raw chopped cashews

  1 tablespoon sesame oil

  ¼ teaspoon sea salt

  6 large collard green leaves

  1 carrot cut into thin matchstick pieces

  1 mango, peeled and cut into thin strips

  1 cup cilantro leaves

  1 cup basil leaves

  ½ cup fresh mint leaves

For the Tamarind Orange Sauce:

  1 cup tamarind pulp

  5 tablespoons fresh squeezed orange juice

  1 tablespoon extra-virgin olive oil

  Pinch of sea salt

Mix the agave, lemon juice, ginger, and soy sauce in a high-speed blender. Then add the almond butter. The consistency should be cakelike. Pour the mixture into a bowl and fold in the shredded cabbage. Mix the cashews, sesame oil, and sea salt in a separate bowl. Cut the center rib away from the collard green leaves. Arrange leaves on a cutting board with underside facing up. Place cabbage mixture, carrots, mango, cilantro, basil, and mint inside the wrap and fold.

To make the sauce, place all ingredients in a high-speed blender and pulse until pureed. Will keep in the refrigerator for up to a week or can also be frozen for up to a month.

SWEET POTATO VEGGIE BURGERS *(8 servings)*

1 large sweet potato

2 teaspoons coconut oil

Two 8-ounce cans cannellini white beans, drained

2 tablespoons tahini

2 teaspoons pure maple syrup or raw agave nectar

1 teaspoon lemon pepper seasoning or Cajun seasoning

1/4 cup wheat flour

3/4 cup panko crumbs

1 tablespoon safflower oil

8 sprouted burger buns

Preheat the oven to 350 degrees. Wash the sweet potato then lightly slit and coat it in coconut oil. Place it in a covered baking dish, bake for about 45 minutes. Peel and place the potato in a large mixing bowl.

Add the beans to the bowl, and mash the potatoes and beans together. Next, mix in the tahini, maple syrup, lemon pepper seasoning, and flour. Your mixture will be quite soft and moist, but you should be able to form a patty. Add more flour to thicken the mixture if needed. Form eight patties from the mixture and coat lightly in panko crumbs. Heat the safflower oil in a pan over high heat.

Place patties in the pan and cook until browned on both sides. You could also bake the burgers. If baking, use 1/2 cup panko and heat the oven to 350 degrees and bake for 25 minutes. Transfer cooked patties to a paper towel. Cool for a few minutes. Serve on toasted sprouted buns with your favorite toppings.

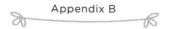

RAW FETTUCCINE WITH SASSY SAGE PESTO *(4 servings)*

This healthy pasta alternative offers a break from the norm. The enzyme-rich raw zucchini helps to clear the colon of buildup, and the sassy sage pesto is earthy and packed with flavor. To slice the zucchini you will need to use a mandolin. Add this peppy pesto to a batch of your favorite pasta, or use it as a spread for sandwiches or as a topping for steamed vegetables or crudités.

> 5 to 6 long straight zucchini
>
> Sassy Sage Pesto (page 243)

Slice the zucchini lengthwise on a mandolin, then slice it again in linguini-width ribbons. Mix the zucchini noodles with the pesto when you are ready to serve, otherwise keep them separate because the salt from the sauce will soften the noodles.

PAN-SEARED TEMPEH *(4 servings)*

> 1 tablespoon freshly grated ginger
>
> 4 tablespoons tamari soy sauce
>
> 1 1/2 tablespoons mirin
>
> 2 teaspoons pure maple syrup
>
> 1/2 teaspoon ground coriander
>
> 2 small garlic cloves, crushed
>
> Juice of 1/2 lime
>
> One 8-ounce package tempeh
>
> 2 tablespoons coconut oil
>
> 1/2 cup chopped cilantro leaves

Mix together the ginger, soy sauce, mirin, maple syrup, coriander, garlic, and lime juice and set aside. Cut the tempeh into thin, bite-sized pieces. Heat the coconut oil in a large frying pan over medium-high heat. When the oil is hot but not smoking, add the tempeh and sear for 5 minutes, or until golden. Turn and cook the other side for another 5 minutes, or until golden. Pour the soy sauce mixture into the pan and simmer for 10 minutes, or until the sauce has reduced to a lovely thick glaze. Garnish with cilantro. Serve hot.

TEAS

DARLING CHAI TEA *(2 servings)*

Chai is one of my favorite drinks. Good for any stage of pregnancy and postpartum, it is earthy, grounding, warm, and soothing. I would pack this tea for myself when traveling and would drink it while breastfeeding as fennel boosts milk production. This is also a great option to alleviate morning sickness.

- 1-inch stick of cinnamon
- 8 cardamom pods
- 1 teaspoon black peppercorns
- 1 tablespoon fennel or anise seed
- 1-inch piece of ginger, grated
- 8 whole cloves
- 1 cup almond milk
- 6 teaspoons raw agave nectar or honey, or to taste
- 3 teaspoons loose white tea or 3 tea bags

Pour 2 cups of water in a small saucepan and add the first six ingredients. Bring the mixture to a boil. Cover, turn heat to low, and simmer for 10 minutes. Add the milk and sweetener and simmer for 5 minutes. Throw in the tea leaves or tea bags, cover, and remove from the heat. After 5 minutes, strain the tea into two cups and serve immediately.

TEA ROYALE: MOROCCAN MINT TEA
WITH ORANGE BLOSSOM WATER *(4 servings)*

I'm inspired by Moroccan cuisine and customs. The high-tea ceremony includes an amazing, fresh mint tea with gunpowder green tea, orange blossom water, and honey. Here I use agave nectar instead. The soothing fresh mint can help ease unsettled stomachs and be a great rejuvenator when energy is low.

1 tablespoon loose Chinese gunpowder green tea leaves

3 to 4 tablespoons raw agave nectar or honey

1 large bunch fresh mint leaves (1 ounce)

1 1/2 tablespoons orange blossom water

Bring 5 cups of water to a boil. Place loose green tea leaves in a teapot and pour in 1 cup boiling water, and then swirl gently to warm pot and rinse tea. Strain out and discard water, reserving tea leaves in pot. Add the remaining 4 cups of boiling water to the tea and let steep for 2 minutes. Stir in the agave nectar and mint and steep for 3 to 4 minutes more. Then add the orange blossom water and stir.

DESSERT

COCONUT ACAI ICE POPS *(8 servings)*

8 ounces acai puree (Sambazon brand)

1/2 cup blueberries

1/2 cup raw agave nectar

1 cup fresh or canned coconut milk

Place the acai puree, blueberries, agave, and 2 cups of water in a high-speed blender and pulse until you have a smooth mixture. Pour about half the mixture into popsicle molds then top off with the coconut milk. Place the popsicle stick inside and freeze for at least 1 hour. Remove popsicles from mold by gently running the molds under warm water.

SASSY CARAMEL POPCORN *(8 servings)*

1 teaspoon coconut oil

½ cup unpopped popcorn kernels

½ cup brown rice syrup

½ cup pure maple syrup

½ teaspoon ground cinnamon

½ teaspoon ground nutmeg

½ teaspoon pure chili powder

½ teaspoon cardamom powder

1 teaspoon fine sea salt

1 cup mixed nuts and seeds (cashews, almonds, pumpkin seeds)

¼ cup dried cranberries

¼ cup dried cherries

Heat the coconut oil in a large heavy pot over high heat. Add the popcorn and cover with a lid. Shake the pan constantly as the kernels start popping to prevent them from burning. Remove from the heat when the popping decreases. Line a baking sheet with parchment paper. In another large pot, bring the syrups, cinnamon, nutmeg, chili powder, cardamom, and salt to a boil over medium heat. As the mixture begins to thicken, add nuts, seeds, berries, and cherries, stirring constantly. Next add the popcorn and mix until well coated. Let stand and cool.

I CAN'T BELIEVE IT'S NOT PUMPKIN PIE *(10 servings)*

This pumpkin pie is actually made with carrot juice, and all the wonderful warming seasonings like nutmeg and cinnamon help to soothe the pancreas and warm the belly. Guess what—no baking required—so this is a great dessert recipe for anyone multitasking in the kitchen, just prep and store in the refrigerator. A great alternative to traditional pumpkin pie, this can be made as a mousse by eliminating the crust.

For the crust:

2 ¼ cups pecans

2 tablespoons pure maple syrup

1 tablespoon coconut oil

1 tablespoon date paste

1 pinch sea salt

For the filling:

½ cup cashews

½ cup pure maple syrup

¼ cups raw agave nectar

½ cup coconut oil

5 ounces carrot juice

½ teaspoon pure vanilla extract

¼ teaspoon sea salt

¼ vanilla bean, split lengthwise and seeds scraped

1 ½ teaspoons ground cinnamon

1 ½ teaspoons ground nutmeg

½ tablespoon chopped thyme

To make the crust, put the pecans in a food processor and pulse until they are small crumbs. Mix the pecans and all the remaining ingredients together by hand. Press mixture into a 9-inch tart pan to the desired thickness. Chill the crust in the freezer for at least an hour.

To make the filling, blend all the ingredients except the thyme in a high-speed blender until very smooth. Stir in the thyme and fill the crust with the mixture. Chill

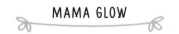
in the freezer for 2 hours, or overnight for best results. Let stand for a half hour at room temperature before serving.

CHOCOLATA CHILI PUDDING *(6 servings)*

Simple to make and a great alternative to all the soy puddings out there. This pudding packs the glow foods coconut and chocolate. Want pudding pops? Just add the mixture to popsicle molds and freeze.

Flesh of 2 to 3 young coconuts

³/₄ cup cocoa powder (Dutch processed)

½ cup pure maple syrup

½ cup raw agave nectar

2 teaspoons pure vanilla extract

3 teaspoons coconut oil

¼ teaspoon sea salt

2 tablespoons ground ancho chili

Blend all ingredients plus 1¹/₃ cups of water in a high-speed blender or food processor until completely smooth. Chill in refrigerator for an hour prior to serving.

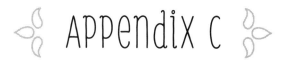

Appendix C

Mama Glow! Resources

Birthing Options/Advocacy

Birth Network National (www.birthnetwork.org): Promoting mother-friendly care.

Childbirth Connection (www.childbirthconnection.org): Helping women and professionals make informed choices.

Choices in Childbirth (choicesinchildbirth.org): The hub for learning about birthing options in NYC, creators of The New York Guide to a Healthy Birth.

Coalition for Improving Maternity Services (www.motherfriendly.org): Promoting a wellness model for maternity care and birth outcomes.

Doulas of North America International (www.dona.org): International certifying body for labor support doulas.

Breastfeeding Support

Ameda (www.ameda.com): Fabulous breast pumps and other feeding products.

La Leche League International (www.lalecheleague.org): Breastfeeding support and advocacy.

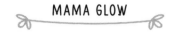

Milkin' Mamas (www.milkinmamas.com): A breast milk donation organization.

Women's Health (www.womenshealth.gov): U.S. Department of Health breastfeeding hotline.

Carriers, Slings, and Strollers

Maclaren Baby (www.maclarenbaby.com): The classic English stroller.

Peppermint (www.peppermint.com): Online destination for baby carriers.

Quinny Stroller (www.quinny.com): Lightweight stroller pick for urban areas.

Stokke (www.stokke.com): Modern sleek stroller design and baby carriers.

Sunshine Baby Slings (www.sunshinebabyslings.com): The most beautiful and practical slings around. Handcrafted with amazing fabrics, they are eco-friendly and durable.

Cesarean Section

Belly Bandit (www.bellybandit.com): Support for your postnatal belly.

Childbirth Connection (www.childbirthconnection.org): Evidence-based research on C-section.

C-Section Recovery (www.csectionrecovery.com): Online resource for speedy recovery from C-section.

International Cesarean Awareness Network (www.ican-online.org): An online community and advocacy resource for cesarean section.

V-BAC (www.vbac.com): Evidence-based info on vaginal birth after cesarean.

Childbirth Education

Birthing From Within (www.birthingfromwithin.com): Pam England's method encouraging women to be powerful in birth.

The Bradley Method (www.bradleybirth.com): Childbirth-education method including prenatal exercise, relaxation, and birth partners as coaches.

Hypnobirthing (www.hypnobirthing.com): A unique childbirth education technique enhanced by hypnosis.

Lamaze International (www.lamaze.org): An international organization promoting a natural approach to pregnancy and childbirth.

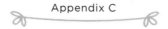

Cleanse and Detox

BE WELL (www.bewellbydrfranklipman.com): Comprehensive science-based cleanse program designed by Dr. Frank Lipman, MD. The *Sustain* formula is great for maintenance for postpartum moms.

BluePrint Cleanse (blueprintcleanse.com): Pressed juice cleanse shipped nationwide.

CLEAN Program (www.cleanprogram.com): Designed by Dr. Alejandro Junger, MD. Clean is a 21-day detox program that supports optimal wellness. Great for cleansing in preparation for conceiving!

One Lucky Duck (www.oneluckyduck.com): Online boutique for all things raw and delicious.

Organic Avenue (www.organicavenue.com): Organic raw vegan juices, raw foods, and supplements shipped nationwide.

RAWvolution (www.rawvolution.com): Matt Amsden's raw food delivery service. So yummy.

Clothing for Baby

Aden & Anais (www.adenandanais.com): Baby brand of organic receiving blankets, swaddles, bedding, and more.

Booda Brand (www.boodabrand.com): Unique kid's T-shirt line from India, inspiring wisdom, wonder, and the will to make a difference.

Bundle (bundlenyc.com): Big style for little ones.

EGG by Susan Lazar (www.egg-baby.com): Organic line of chic baby apparel.

G-Diapers (www.gdiapers.com): Reusable, biodegradable diapers.

Kate Quinn Organics (www.katequinnorganics.com): Natural luxury line for babies.

Clothing for Mama

Fit 2 B Mom (www.fit2Bmom.com): Hip maternity workout duds for the fit and active mama.

Hatch Collection (hatchcollection.com): A collection of chic, timeless, and cozy wardrobe essentials for before, during, and after pregnancy.

Isabella Oliver (www.isabellaoliver.com): Luxurious maternity pieces for women who love clothes.

Unbuttoned Maternity (www.unbuttonedmaternity.com): Ultra-chic maternity boutique.

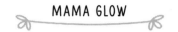
Vanessa Knox Maternity (www.vanessaknox.com): High-end elegant maternity garments for ultra-chic occasions and everyday affairs.

Victoria Keen Designs (www.v-keen.com): Beautiful hand-silk-screened clothing made in NYC.

Concierge Services

The Baby Planners (www.thebabyplanners.com): The nation's premier baby concierge and consulting company.

It's a Belly (www.itsabelly.com): Maternity concierge, baby planners for your belly and beyond.

Premier Baby Concierge (premierbabyconcierge.com): Preparing you for a bundle of new experiences.

Sissy & Marley (sissyandmarley.com): Boutique concierge services for the birth journey.

Sweet Pea Baby Planners (www.sweetpeababyplanners.com): Full pre/postnatal concierge with locations across the country.

CSA Community Supported Agriculture and Organic Food

Farmers' Market (www.farmersmarket.com): Online resource to find your local farmers, market.

Food Routes (www.foodroutes.org): Education and advocacy site for locally grown food.

Local Harvest (www.localharvest.org/csa): Resource for buying local, supporting CSAs, and food events.

Organic (www.organic.org): Organic made easy. Life made better. An educational resource for organics.

Sustainable Table (www.sustainabletable.org): Serving up healthy food choices in education and advocacy around local and sustainable foodstuffs.

Eco-Boutiques

Eco Mom (www.ecomom.com): A destination site for eco-friendly products for moms and their little ones.

The Little Seed (www.thelittleseed.com): L.A.-based hip children's boutique carrying eco-friendly organic products.

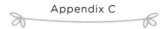

The WellNEST (wellnest.us): Hamptons-based eco-lifestyle boutique and vitamin store for holistic living and home décor.

Herbal Support

Chakra 4 Herbal Apothecary (www.chakra4herbs.com): High-quality herbs from around the world.

H. Gillerman Organics (www.hgillermanorganics.com): Pure crafted essential oil blends for optimal health.

Jurlique (www.jurlique.com): Balancing essential oils and botanicals.

Young Living Essential Oils (www.youngliving.com): High-quality essential oils.

Online Communities and Resources

The Bump (www.thebump.com): Guide to your pregnancy.

Café Mom (www.cafemom.com): A meeting place for moms.

Ecomii (www.ecomii.com): Comprehensive resource for green living.

Giggle (www.giggle.com): Lifestyle destination for pregnancy and parenthood.

Hollywood Hot Moms (www.hollywoodhotmoms.com): Jessica Denay's online resource for hip moms and moms-to-be.

Lifetime Moms (www.lifetimemoms.com): Real life. Real women. Real stories.

Modern Mom (www.modernmom.com): Brooke Burke's lifestyle hub for pregnancy and parenting.

Mom Bloggers Club (www.mombloggersclub.com): Connect with thousands of mom bloggers.

My Best Birth (www.mybestbirth.com): Ricki Lake and Abby Epstein's birth community.

Naturally Savvy (www.naturallysavvy.com): Organic lifestyle destination.

5 Minutes for Mom (www.5minutesformom.com): A blogging community for moms.

Skin Care/Beauty

Basq Skin Care (www.basqnyc.com): Upscale maternity skin-care line.

Belli Skin Care (www.belliskincare.com): Pregnancy, motherhood, and baby skin care.

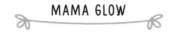
Belly Vita (www.bellyvita.com): Creators of Belly Imprint™ Spa treatment and Sculpting Kit.

Burt's Bees (www.burtsbees.com): Natural skin care for mothers and babies.

Carol's Daughter (www.carolsdaughter.com): Luxury natural skin- and hair-care line for women of color.

Earth Mama Angel Baby (www.earthmamaangelbaby.com): Herbal-based skin- and self-care line for mothers and babies.

Erba Viva (www.erbaviva.com): Botanically inspired upscale skin-care line for mothers and babies.

Georgia (www.georgiany.com): A mother's luxury skin care for every day.

Little Twig (www.littletwig.com): Eco-bath-and-body line for baby and mommy.

Pangea Organics (www.pangeaorganics.com): Organic and eco-centric body care for the family.

Raw Gaia (www.rawgaia.com): Raw skin care that's good for you and the planet.

Tata Harper Skin Care (www.tataharperskincare.com): Superior botanical skin-care line for mother's face and body.

Vapour Organic Beauty (www.vapourbeauty.com): Organic and cruelty-free makeup and beauty products.

Weleda Skin Care (usa.weleda.com): Botanical skin care for babies and moms.

Vegan Lifestyle

Crazy Sexy Life (crazysexylife.com): Author and cancer survivor Kris Carr's whimsical website and blog that is all about embracing healthy eating and mindful living.

Earth Cafe To-Go (earthcafetogo.com): Raw cheesecakes, with no dairy, gluten, or sugar. Eleven different delightful flavors.

Girlie Girl Army (girliegirlarmy.com): Your Glamazon guide to green living and a vegan lifestyle. Powered by Mama Glow Icon Chloé Jo Davis.

Nibmor Chocolates (www.nibmor.com): Raw organic, vegan, handcrafted chocolate bars.

PETA—People for the Ethical Treatment of Animals (www.peta.org): A vegan organization dedicated to protecting the rights of animals.

VegNews (vegnews.com): An award-winning vegan magazine with recipes, travel, food, and news.

Yoga Lifestyle

Gaiam (www.gaiam.com): A holistic lifestyle hub and community that also sells mats, props, products, apparel, and videos.

Hyde (yogahyde.com): Conscious, comfortable, and cute yoga wear for all.

Lululemon (www.lululemon.com): High-end yoga apparel, gear, mats, and props.

Manduka (www.manduka.com): My favorite yoga products.

Yoga Journal (www.yogajournal.com): Print and online support for your yoga practice.

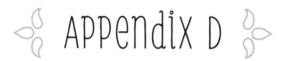

Appendix D

Blissful Birth Plan

Full name:

Partner's name:

Today's date:

Due date OR induction date:

Doctor's name:

Hospital name:

Please note that I: [ ] Have group B strep [ ] Am Rh incompatible with the baby [ ] Have gestational diabetes

My delivery is planned as: [ ] Vaginal [ ] C-section [ ] Water birth [ ] VBAC

I'd like . . . :

[ ] Partner:
[ ] Parents:
[ ] Other children:
[ ] Doula:
[ ] Other:

present before AND/OR during labor

During labor, I'd like: [ ] Music played (I will provide) [ ] The lights dimmed [ ] The room as quiet as possible [ ] As few interruptions as possible [ ] As few vaginal exams as possible [ ] Hospital staff limited to my own doctor and nurses (no students, residents, or interns present) [ ] To wear my own clothes [ ] To wear my contact lenses the entire time [ ] My partner to film AND/OR take pictures [ ] My partner to be present the entire time [ ] To stay hydrated with clear liquids and ice chips [ ] To eat and drink as approved by my doctor

I'd like to spend the first stage of labor: [ ] Standing up [ ] Lying down [ ] Walking around [ ] In the shower [ ] In the bathtub

I'd like to spend early labor: [ ] At home [ ] Settling in at place of delivery

I'm not interested in: [ ] An enema [ ] Shaving of my pubic area [ ] A urinary catheter [ ] An IV, unless I'm dehydrated (and a Heparin or saline lock IS/IS NOT ok)

I'd like fetal monitoring to be: [ ] Continuous [ ] Intermittent [ ] Internal [ ] External [ ] Performed only by Doppler [ ] Performed only if the baby is in distress

I'd like labor augmentation: [ ] Performed only if the baby is in distress [ ] First attempted by natural methods such as nipple stimulation [ ] Performed by membrane stripping [ ] Performed with prostaglandin gel [ ] Performed with Pitocin [ ] Performed by rupture of the membrane [ ] Performed by stripping of the membrane [ ] Never to include an artificial rupture of the membrane

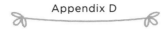

For pain relief, I'd like to use: [ ] Acupressure [ ] Acupuncture [ ] Breathing techniques [ ] Cold therapy [ ] Demerol [ ] Distraction [ ] Hot therapy [ ] Hypnosis [ ] Massage [ ] Meditation [ ] Reflexology [ ] Standard epidural [ ] TENS [ ] Walking epidural [ ] Nothing [ ] Only what I request at the time [ ] Whatever is suggested at the time

During delivery, I would like to: [ ] Squat [ ] Semi-recline [ ] Lie on my side [ ] Be on my hands and knees [ ] Stand [ ] Lean on my partner [ ] Use people for leg support [ ] Use foot pedals for support [ ] Use a birth bar for support [ ] Use a birthing stool [ ] Be in a birthing tub [ ] Be in the shower

I will bring a: [ ] Birthing ball [ ] Birthing chair [ ] Squatting bar [ ] Birthing tub

As the baby is delivered, I would like to: [ ] Push spontaneously [ ] Push as directed [ ] Push without time limits, as long as the baby and I are not at risk [ ] Use a mirror to see the baby crown [ ] Touch the head as it crowns [ ] Let the epidural wear off while pushing [ ] Have a full dose of epidural [ ] Avoid forceps usage [ ] Avoid vacuum extraction [ ] Use whatever methods my doctor deems necessary [ ] Help catch the baby [ ] Let my partner catch the baby [ ] Let my partner suction the baby

I would like an episiotomy: [ ] Performed only as a last resort [ ] Used only after perineal massage, warm compresses, and positioning [ ] Rather than risk a tear [ ] Not performed, even if it means risking a tear [ ] Performed as medically necessary [ ] Performed with local anesthesia [ ] Followed by local anesthesia for the repair

Immediately after delivery, I would like: [ ] My partner to cut the umbilical cord [ ] The umbilical cord to be cut only after it stops pulsating [ ] To bank the cord blood [ ] To donate the cord blood [ ] To deliver the placenta spontaneously and without assistance [ ] To see the placenta before it is discarded [ ] Not to be given Pitocin/oxytocin

If a C-section is necessary, I would like: [ ] A second opinion [ ] To make sure all other options have been exhausted [ ]To stay conscious [ ] My partner to remain with me the entire time [ ] The screen lowered so I can watch the baby come out [ ] My hands left free so I can touch the baby [ ] The surgery explained as it

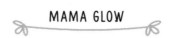

happens [ ] An epidural for anesthesia [ ] My partner to hold the baby as soon as possible [ ] To breastfeed ASAP in the recovery room

I would like to hold the baby: [ ] Immediately after delivery [ ] After suctioning [ ] After weighing [ ] After being wiped clean and swaddled [ ] Before eye drops/ointment are given

I would like to breastfeed: [ ] As soon as possible after delivery [ ] Before eye drops/ointment are given [ ] Later [ ] Never

I'd like my family members (NAMES):

[ ] To join me and the baby immediately after delivery [ ] To join me and the baby in the room later [ ] Only to see the baby in the nursery [ ] To have unlimited visiting after birth

I'd like the baby's medical exam and procedures: [ ] Given in my presence [ ] Given only after we've bonded [ ] Given in my partner's presence [ ] To include a heel stick for screening tests beyond the PKU [ ] To include a hearing screening test [ ] To include a hepatitis B vaccine

Please don't give the baby: [ ] Vitamin K [ ] Antibiotic eye treatment [ ] Sugar water [ ] Formula [ ] A pacifier

I'd like the baby's first bath given: [ ] In my presence [ ] In my partner's presence [ ] By me [ ] By my partner

I'd like to feed the baby: [ ] Only with breast milk [ ] Only with formula [ ] On demand [ ] On schedule [ ] With the help of a lactation specialist

I'd like the baby to stay in my room: [ ] All the time [ ] During the day [ ] Only when I'm awake [ ] Only for feeding [ ] Only when I request

I'd like my partner: [ ] To have unlimited visiting [ ] To sleep in my room

If we have a boy, circumcision should: [ ] Be performed [ ] Not be performed [ ] Be performed later [ ] Be performed with anesthesia [ ] Be performed in the presence of me AND/OR my partner

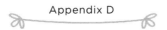

As needed post-delivery, please give me: [ ] Extra-strength acetaminophen [ ] Percocet [ ] Stool softener [ ] Laxative [ ] Water

After birth, I'd like to stay in the hospital: [ ] As long as possible [ ] As briefly as possible

If the baby is not well, I'd like: [ ] My partner and I to accompany it to the NICU or another facility [ ] To breastfeed or provide pumped breast milk [ ] To hold him or her whenever possible

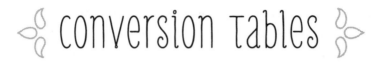

conversion tables

Standard Cup	Fine Powder (e.g., flour)	Grain (e.g., rice)	Granular (e.g., sugar)	Liquid Solids (e.g., butter)	Liquid (e.g., milk)
1	140 g	150 g	190 g	200 g	240 ml
³/₄	105 g	113 g	143 g	150 g	180 ml
²/₃	93 g	100 g	125 g	133 g	160 ml
¹/₂	70 g	75 g	95 g	100 g	120 ml
¹/₃	47 g	50 g	63 g	67 g	80 ml
¹/₄	35 g	38 g	48 g	50 g	60 ml
¹/₈	18 g	19 g	24 g	25 g	30 ml

Useful Equivalents for Liquid Ingredients by Volume					
¹/₄ tsp				1 ml	
¹/₂ tsp				2 ml	
1 tsp				5 ml	
3 tsp	1 tbsp		¹/₂ fl oz	15 ml	
	2 tbsp	¹/₈ cup	1 fl oz	30 ml	
	4 tbsp	¹/₄ cup	2 fl oz	60 ml	
	5 ¹/₃ tbsp	¹/₃ cup	3 fl oz	80 ml	
	8 tbsp	¹/₂ cup	4 fl oz	120 ml	
	10 ²/₃ tbsp	²/₃ cup	5 fl oz	160 ml	
	12 tbsp	³/₄ cup	6 fl oz	180 ml	
	16 tbsp	1 cup	8 fl oz	240 ml	
	1 pt	2 cups	16 fl oz	480 ml	
	1 qt	4 cups	32 fl oz	960 ml	
			33 fl oz	1000 ml	1 l

Useful Equivalents for Dry Ingredients by Weight		
To convert ounces to grams, multiply the number of ounces by 30.		
1 oz	$^1/_{16}$ lb	30 g
4 oz	$^1/_4$ lb	120 g
8 oz	$^1/_2$ lb	240 g
12 oz	$^3/_4$ lb	360 g
16 oz	1 lb	480 g

Useful Equivalents for Cooking/Oven Temperatures			
Process	Fahrenheit	Celsius	Gas Mark
Freeze Water	32° F	0° C	
Room Temperature	68° F	20° C	
Boil Water	212° F	100° C	
Bake	325° F	160° C	3
	350° F	180° C	4
	375° F	190° C	5
	400° F	200° C	6
	425° F	220° C	7
	450° F	230° C	8
Broil			Grill

Useful Equivalents for Length				
To convert inches to centimeters, multiply the number of inches by 2.5.				
1 in			2.5 cm	
6 in	$^1/_2$ ft		15 cm	
12 in	1 ft		30 cm	
36 in	3 ft	1 yd	90 cm	
40 in			100 cm	1 m

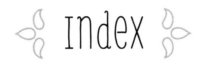

Index

Index of Recipes

Agave nectar, 78
Algaes, 237
Apples
    Butternut Squash Apple Soup, 284
    Green Juice, 262
    The Mama Blood Builder, 35
    Skin Food Juice, 262
Apricot Milk, 261
Artichoke Hearts, Fava Beans, and Shitake Salad, 172
Avocados
    about: breastfeeding benefits of, 237
    Avocado, Watercress & Cumin Salad, 268
    Carrot Avocado Sun Soup, 282
    Low-Fat Guacamole, 266
    Mama's Mango-Avo-Serrano Relish, 276

Bananas
    Blackberry Cream Smoothie, 259
    Cherry Banana Split Smoothie, 176
    Tunisian Plantains, 291
Basil, in Sassy Sage Pesto, 241
Beans and legumes. See also Soy products
    about: breastfeeding benefits of, 238; go-to glow foods, 83; sprouting, 128–129
    Artichoke Hearts, Fava Beans, and Shitake Salad, 172
    Black-Eyed Pea Dip, 265
    Brazil Nuts with Sun-Dried Tomatoes & Bean Salad, 268
    Easy Peasy Sprouts, 129
    Garlic Ginger Green Beans, 174
    Jalapeño Hummus, 292
    Low-Fat Guacamole, 266
    Mexi-Cali Black Beans, 294
    Spicy Chickpea & Lentil Soup, 280

Beets, in Smooth Operator, 263
Berries
    about: breastfeeding benefits of, 237–238; goji berries, 23
    Acai & Blueberry Omega Protein Blast, 257
    Blackberry Cream Smoothie, 259
    Coconut Acai Ice Pops, 301
    Cranberry Balsamic Brussels Sprouts, 286
    Cranberry-Curry Couscous in a Hurry, 287
    Wild Blueberry & Hemp Shake, 258
Boob foods, 235–241
    about: Brazil Nut Milk, 240; breakfasts, lunches, dinners, snacks, 238–239; categories of, 236–238; coconut milk, 240; hemp milk, 240; weaning and, 239–240
    Brazil Nut Milk, 240
    Rockstar Granola, 236
    Sassy Sage Pesto, 241
Breads
    about: flour types, 129–130
    Coconut Chapatis, 295
    Green Chili Cornbread, 293
Breakfast recipes
    Breakfast Polenta Recipe, 264
    Quinoa Porridge, 263
Brussels sprouts, cranberry balsamic, 286
Butternut Squash Apple Soup, 284

Cabbage, in Not Your Grandma's Coleslaw Salad, 273
Cacao. See Chocolate and cacao
Carrots
    Cardamom Carrot Salad, 270
    Carrot Avocado Sun Soup, 282
    Carrot Cumin Dip, 264
    Not Your Grandma's Coleslaw Salad, 273
    Raw Hearty Chunky Chili, 283
    Snack Mix, 266
Chai tea, 300

Chapatis, coconut, 295
Cheese alternatives, 27
Cherry Banana Split Smoothie, 176
Chickpeas. *See* Beans and legumes
Chili, 283
Chocolate and cacao
  about: cacao, 23; pleasure and benefits of, 175
  Cacao Breeze Smoothie, 259
  Chocolata Chili Pudding, 304
Citrus
  about: acidic flavorings, 86
  Coco-Lime Smoothie, 259
  Lemon-Fennel-Olive Relish, 277
  Lemon Tahini Dressing, 275
  Tamarind Orange Sauce, 297–298
  Tea Royale: Moroccan Mint Tea with Orange
    Blossom Water, 301
Coconut
  about: milk, 240; nectar, 78
  Chocolata Chili Pudding, 304
  Coco-Lime Smoothie, 259
  Coconut Acai Ice Pops, 301
  Coconut Chapatis, 295
Coffee, in Latham's Coffee Sugar Scrub, 149
Collard Wraps with Tamarind Orange Sauce,
  297–298
Comfort foods
  Artichoke Hearts, Fava Beans, and Shitake
    Salad, 172
  Cherry Banana Split Smoothie, 176
  Garlic Ginger Green Beans, 174
  Watermelon Diva Salad, 173
Corn and polenta
  Breakfast Polenta Recipe, 264
  Green Chili Cornbread, 293
  Sassy Caramel Popcorn, 302
  Sweet Baby Corn Relish, 278
  Sweet Lemongrass and Lime Corn, 290
Couscous, cranberry-curry, 287
Cucumbers
  Gazpacho, 285
  Skin Food Juice, 262

Desserts
  about: sugar alternatives, 77–78; sweetening
    ingredients, 88
  Chocolata Chili Pudding, 304
  Coconut Acai Ice Pops, 301
  I Can't Believe It's Not Pumpkin Pie, 303–304
  Rice Pudding Pick-Me-Up, 226
  Sassy Caramel Popcorn, 302
  Vanilla Chia Pudding, 59
Dill dressing, 275
Dips and spreads. *See* Snacks
Dressings
  Goddess Herb Dressing, 82
  Lemon Tahini Dressing, 275
  Luscious Dill Dressing, 275
  Rich Garlic Dressing, 274
  Sun-Dried Tomato Vinaigrette, 274
Drinks. *See also* Smoothies and juices
  about: avoiding dehydration, 68–69, 162;
    Brazil nut milk, 240; caffeine alternatives, 24;
    coconut milk, 240; hemp milk, 240; nut milk
    bags, 85; nut milks, 27, 240, 260; water intake,

17–18, 68–69
  Apricot Milk, 261
  Basic Almond Milk, 28
  Basic Nut Milk Recipe, 260
  Brazil Nut Milk, 240
  Darling Chai Tea, 300
  Fertili-Tea, 13
  Instant Cashew-Hemp Milk, 261
  Lavender-Ginger Goddess Tonic, 55
  The Mama Blood Builder, 35
  Tea Royale: Moroccan Mint Tea with Orange
    Blossom Water, 301

Entrées
  Collard Wraps with Tamarind Orange Sauce,
    297–298
  Pan-Seared Tempeh, 299
  Raw Fettuccine with Sassy Sage Pesto, 299
  Sweet Potato Veggie Burgers, 298
  Vegan Moroccan Tagine, 296–297

Fats and oils, 21–22, 72–73, 86–87
Fruits
  about: breastfeeding benefits of, 237–238;
    dried, 88; fatty, 86; go-to glow foods, 83; raw,
    63–64

Garlic
  Garlic Ginger Green Beans, 174
  Rich Garlic Dressing, 274
  Tomato & Garlic Salad, 271
Ginger, in Lavender-Ginger Goddess Tonic, 55
Glow foods. *See General Index*
Grains. *See also* Breads; Quinoa
  about: flour types, 129–130; gluten-free whole
    grains, 236; gluten sensitivity, 130–131; go-to
    glow foods, 83; storing, 63–64; wheat, 130–131
  Cranberry-Curry Couscous in a Hurry, 287
  Rockstar Granola, 236
  Snack Mix, 266
  Sprouted Tabbouleh, 288
Green beans, garlic ginger, 174
Greens. *See also* Salads
  about: breastfeeding benefits of, 237; go-to
    glow foods, 83; minerals in, 66; nutritional
    benefits, 65–66, 237; vitamin K and, 66
  Collard Wraps with Tamarind Orange Sauce,
    297–298
  Green Juice, 262
  Juice It!, 220
  Sassy Sautéed Collard Green Ribbons, 67

Hemp. *See* Nuts and seeds
Honey, 78, 88
Hummus, 292

Ingredients. *See also specific main ingredients*
  acidic flavorings, 86
  glow foods. *See General Index*
  healthy fats, 86–87
  omgega-3s, 72–73
  pantry items to stock, 86–88
  savory and salty, 87
  stocking pantry and refrigerator, 165
  sweet, 87

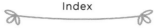

Juices. *See* Smoothies and juices

Kale
    Green Juice, 262
    Juice It!, 220
    The Mama Blood Builder, 35
    Rockin' Kale d, 269
    Tunisian Kale Salad, 272

Lavender-Ginger Goddess Tonic, 55
Lentils. *See* Beans and legumes

Maca, 23
Macadamia Nut Sour Cream, 279
Mangoes
    Mama's Mango-Avo-Serrano Relish, 276
    Pineapple-Mango Salsa, 279
Maple syrup, 78
Milks. *See* Drinks
Mushrooms
    Artichoke Hearts, Fava Beans, and Shitake
      Salad, 172
    Magic Mushroom Soup, 281

Nuts and seeds
    about: Brazil nut milk, 240; buying, 86–87; go-to
      glow foods, 83; hemp milk, 240; hemp seeds,
      23; nut milk bags, 85; nut milks, 27, 240, 260;
      nut/nut-butter fats, 86–87; raw, 63–64; seed
      nutrition, 237; for skin care, 151; soaking, 128;
      sprouting, 128–129; stocking, 86–87; storing,
      63–64
    Almond Joy Smoothie, 258
    Apricot Milk, 261
    Basic Almond Milk, 28
    Basic Nut Milk Recipe, 260
    Brazil Nut Milk, 240
    Brazil Nuts with Sun-Dried Tomatoes & Bean
      Salad, 268
    Coco-Lime Smoothie, 259
    Easy Peasy Sprouts, 129
    I Can't Believe It's Not Pumpkin Pie, 303–304
    Instant Cashew-Hemp Milk, 261
    Macadamia Nut Sour Cream, 279
    Raw Hearty Chunky Chili, 283
    Raw Sesame-Coated Majoun, 267
    Rockstar Granola, 236
    Snack Mix, 266
    Vanilla Chia Pudding, 59
    Wild Blueberry & Hemp Shake, 258

Pasta, Raw Fettuccine with Sassy Sage Pesto, 299
Pears
    Blackberry Cream Smoothie, 259
    Pear Protein Smoothie, 256
Peppers
    Gazpacho, 285
    Green Chili Cornbread, 293
    Mama's Mango-Avo-Serrano Relish, 276
Pesto, 241
Pineapple
    Pineapple-Mango Salsa, 279
    Skin Food Juice, 262
    Smooth Operator, 263

Pineapple-Mango Salsa, 279
Plantains, Tunisian, 291
Polenta, breakfast recipe, 264
Pumpkin-pie-like dessert, 303–304

Quinoa
    Inca Protein Queen Salad, 75
    Quinoa Porridge, 263

Recipes, overview of this book and, xx–xxi, 255
Relishes, salsas, and creams
    Lemon-Fennel-Olive Relish, 277
    Macadamia Nut Sour Cream, 279
    Mama's Mango-Avo-Serrano Relish, 276
    Pico de Gallo, 279
    Pineapple-Mango Salsa, 279
    Sweet Baby Corn Relish, 278
    Tamarind Orange Sauce, 297–298
Rice
    about: brown rice benefits, 238; brown rice
      syrup, 78
    Rice Pudding Pick-Me-Up, 226

Salads
    Artichoke Hearts, Fava Beans, and Shitake
      Salad, 172
    Avocado, Watercress & Cumin Salad, 268
    Brazil Nuts with Sun-Dried Tomatoes & Bean
      Salad, 268
    Cardamom Carrot Salad, 270
    Inca Protein Queen Salad, 75
    Not Your Grandma's Coleslaw Salad, 273
    Rockin' Kale Salad, 269
    Tomato & Garlic Salad, 271
    Tunisian Kale Salad, 272
    Watermelon Diva Salad, 173
Salsas. *See* Relishes, salsas, and creams
Salt and salty ingredients, 87
Savory ingredients, 87
Seeds. *See* Nuts and seeds
Side dishes
    Coconut Chapatis, 295
    Cranberry Balsamic Brussels Sprouts, 286
    Cranberry-Curry Couscous in a Hurry, 287
    Gingerly Mashed Sweet Potatoes with Lime,
      289
    Green Chili Cornbread, 293
    Jalapeño Hummus, 292
    Mexi-Cali Black Beans, 294
    Sprouted Tabbouleh, 288
    Sweet Lemongrass and Lime Corn, 290
    Tunisian Plantains, 291
Skin care recipes
    about: healthy breakfast augmenting, 148
    Anointing Body Butter, 147
    Hydrating Facial Masque, 149
    Latham's Coffee Sugar Scrub, 149
    Stretch Mark Prevention Oil, 151
    Tata Harper's Face/Body Scrub, 148
Smoothies and juices
    about: juicers/juice extractors, 84
    Acai & Blueberry Omega Protein Blast, 257
    Almond Joy Smoothie, 258
    Basic Smoothie, 256
    Blackberry Cream Smoothie, 259

Cacao Breeze Smoothie, 259
Cherry Banana Split Smoothie, 176
Goji Sunset Smoothie, 257
Green Juice, 262
Juice It!, 220
Pear Protein Smoothie, 256
Skin Food Juice, 262
Smooth Operator, 263
Wild Blueberry & Hemp Shake, 258
Snacks
    Black-Eyed Pea Dip, 265
    Carrot Cumin Dip, 264
    Edamame Spread, 265
    Low-Fat Guacamole, 266
    Raw Sesame-Coated Majoun, 267
    Snack Mix, 266
Soups
    Butternut Squash Apple Soup, 284
    Carrot Avocado Sun Soup, 282
    Gazpacho, 285
    Magic Mushroom Soup, 281
    Raw Hearty Chunky Chili, 283
    Spicy Chickpea & Lentil Soup, 280
Soy products
    about: pros and cons of, 22
    Black-Eyed Pea Dip, 265
    Edamame Spread, 265
Spirulina, 22–23
Spreads and dips. See Snacks
Sprouts
    Easy Peasy Sprouts, 129
    Sprouted Tabbouleh, 288
Stevia, 78
Sweet potatoes
    Cumin-Cinnamon Roasted Sweet Potatoes, 79
    Gingerly Mashed Sweet Potatoes with Lime, 289
    Sweet Potato Veggie Burgers, 298

Tamarind Orange Sauce, 297–298
Teas
    Darling Chai Tea, 300
    Fertili-Tea, 13
    Tea Royale: Moroccan Mint Tea with Orange Blossom Water, 301
Tempeh
    Pan-Seared Tempeh, 299
    Vegan Moroccan Tagine, 296–297
Tomatoes
    Brazil Nuts with Sun-Dried Tomatoes & Bean Salad, 268
    Gazpacho, 285
    Pico de Gallo, 279
    Raw Hearty Chunky Chili, 283
    Tomato & Garlic Salad, 271

Vanilla Chia Pudding, 59
Vegetables
    about: go-to glow foods, 83; importance of eating, 19–20; nutritional benefits, 19; raw, 63–64; sea vegetables, 20, 83
Veggie burgers, 298

Watermelon Diva Salad, 173

Yacon syrup, 78

General Index

Acidic flavorings, 86
Affirmations
    defined, 37
    for inner guidance, 100–102
    for radical self-care, 248
    for self-love, 105
ALA (alpha linolenic acid), 73
Algaes, 237
Alpha waves, 168
Antioxidants
    eating fruits and vegetables for, 233
    oxidants and, 17
    recipes featuring, 35, 257, 258, 268
    strongest on planet, 23
    super-foods with, 15–16, 23, 237–238
    vitamins as, 17, 24
Appetite, supplement for, 54
Atkins diet, 131
Awkward Chair Pose, 138

Baby
    attitude toward, 199
    birth of. See Birth; Contractions; Labor
    kissing connection with, 235
    sacred pact with, 53
    skin-to-skin contact, 207, 222
Baby blues and PPD, 222–225
Baby clothes and supplies, 166
Baby development
    first trimester, 52
    second trimester, 110
    third trimester, 158
Baggage, unloading, 7–9
Bathing, 20–21, 60, 159, 160, 163, 217, 250
Beauty essentials, 145–154. See also Skin care
    about: overview of, 145–146
    Glow kit and tips, 153
    hair care, 152, 209
Beliefs, limiting, cleansing, 8–9
Beta waves, 168
Binn, Haley, 209
Birth. See also Contractions; Labor
    childbirth education resources, 306–307
    C-section, 205, 306
    episiotomies, 205–206
    hormone cocktail party of, 194–197
    at hospital, 117–118
    immediately after, 207
    induction, 204
    location options, 117–118, 305
    natural vs. pain management, 119–120. See also Epidural anesthesia
    nesting to-dos before, 164–166
    no separation after, 207
    optimal positions for, 200
    planning for the unplanned, 203–206
    P.U.S.H. approach, 206–207
    sexual activity before, 166–167, 189. See also Orgasms
    skin-to-skin contact after, 207, 222
    slow, 142–143
    soundscape/playlist for, 193–194
    who-to-call list, 166

Birth announcements, 165
Birth bag basics, 191–193
Birth centers, 117, 118
Birth coaches (doulas), 118, 143, 186–188
Birth plan
    overview, 185
    template, 313–317
Birth room, 166–167
Bladder, increased urination, 56–57
Blenders, 84
Blood sugar, balancing, 16, 66, 121–122, 130, 188. *See also* Insulin
Boat Pose, 245
Body (yours)
    cleansing, 9–10
    increased urination, 56–57
    learning to appreciate, 11
    listening to, 51–52
    loving, 47, 104–106
    new, after pregnancy, 243–245
    orgasms and, 46–47, 99, 167, 168, 180, 196
    overheating, 53
    preparing for labor, 158–160
    sacred anatomy, 103–106
    self-love affirmations, 105
    sexual organs, 103–104
    "womb-iverse" and, 10–11
Boob foods, 235–241
Book overview, xiv–xv, xix–xxii, 251–252
Brain health, 23, 73
Brain waves, 168
Braxton-Hicks contractions, 157, 159
Breakfast
    about: breastfeeding and, 238; healthy, for skin health, 148
    Glimmer detox, 32, 33
    Glitz detox, 30, 31
    Glow detox, 34
    recipes for. *See Index of Recipes*
Breastfeeding
    baby immune system and, 232
    benefits and challenges, 214–215, 232
    breast development before, 110
    classes and support, 188, 214
    formula alternatives, 234–235
    GLA oils and, 216
    hands-free, 227
    latching challenges, 218–219
    let-down reflex, 215–216
    maintaining milk production, 232–234
    mastitis and, 219–220
    oxytocin and, 203, 215, 232
    skin-to-skin contact and, 207, 222
    support resources, 305–306
    thrush and, 221–222
    weaning baby from, 239–240
Breasts
    boob foods for, 235–241
    engorgement of, 216–217
    inflammation of (mastitis), 219–220
    pain relief, 216–217
    saline solution bath, 222
Breathing
    awareness states and, 93–94
    deep, effects of, 48

meditation and, 94
    practicing, 94–95
    relaxing pelvic floor, 94, 167
    sound, opening and, 98–100
Bridge, supported pose, 184
Brower, Elena, 48
B vitamins. *See* Vitamin B (B vitamins)

Caffeine alternatives, 24
Calcium, 26, 66, 70, 72, 74, 116, 162, 175, 233
Call list, for birth announcement, 166
Carbohydrates, complex, 70, 76–77, 130
Carriers, 306
Carr, Kris, 19
Cat posture, 137, 138–139
Cesarean sections, 205, 306
Checklists, 89, 102, 208
Cheese cloth, 85
Child's Pose, 43
Chinois, 84
Chlorella, 237
Chocolate. *See Index of Recipes*
Cleansing
    blocks to creativity, 11
    clutter, 4–5
    limiting beliefs, 8–9
    resources, 307
    weeding out whackness, 11–12
    "womb-iverse" and, 10–11
    your body, 9–10
Clearance, making
    about, 37
    affirmations and, 37
    movement meditation, 38–39
    planting seeds of renewal, 39
    practicing, 38
    womb-ifestation meditation, 39–40
    yoga plan, 40–41
Clothing, resources, 307–308
Clutter
    clearing out, 4–5, 47–48
    home reflecting inner world and, 4
Cobbler's Pose (Shakti Seat), 96
Colorful foods, 68
Combining foods, 125
Comfort foods, 171–176
    chocolate, 175
    recipes, 172–174, 176
    therapeutic foods vs., 127
Conception. *See* Preparing to conceive
Concierge services, 308
Consciousness, brain waves and, 168
Constipation, 115–116
Contractions
    after birth, 203
    Braxton-Hicks, 157, 159
    F.E.A.R. and, 197–198
    frequency of, 201–202
    nipple stimulation and, 167
    oxytocin initiating, 195
    phone app. timer, 192
    premature, 69, 72, 159–160
    sound, opening and, 98–100, 167
Cooking food
    dehydrating and, 128

fermenting and, 128
food combining and, 125
foundation, balance and, 126
gratitude, attitude and, 126
guidelines, 124–125
intention and, 126
intuitively, 126
as meditation, 124
mindful principles, 125–127
preparation methods, 127–129
preparing to, 124
protein intake and, 131–132
in quantity, 164–165
restaurant food vs., 123–124
sensual preparation, 126–127
soaking and, 128
sprouting and, 128–129
therapeutic vs. comfort foods, 127
Cookware, green, 85
Cow posture, 137, 138–139
Cramps, leg, 162–163
Cravings, 57–61
attitude toward, 58
benefits of, 58
causes of, 57–58
decoder chart, 61
deconstructing, 59–61
pudding recipe for, 59

Dairy, 25–28
alternatives to, 27–28
cow's milk drawbacks, 25–27
sugar in, 27
vitamin D and, 26
Dancing, 163, 244
Dehydrating food
dehydrators for, 84
process of, 128
Dehydration, 68–69, 162
Delta waves, 168
Detox. See Glow guidelines; Prepregnancy detox
Development by trimester. See Trimester references
DHA, 73
Diabetes, gestational, 121–122
Diet. See Cleansing; Cooking food; Food and nutrition; Glow foods; Vitamins and minerals
Digestion
mindful eating practices and, 132–133
reflux/indigestion/heartburn, 113–115
sluggish bowels/constipation, 115–116
Dilation, of cervix, 168, 200–201
Dinner
about: breastfeeding and, 239
Glimmer detox, 32–33
Glitz detox, 31
Glow detox, 34
recipes for. See Index of Recipes
DMT, 196, 203
Doulas, 118, 143, 186–188
"Dove Pose", 182–183
Dove Series, 141
Downward-Dog Plies, 245
Downward-Dog Split, 42
Downward-Facing Dog, 43, 138, 141, 183

Earth Rooting Pose (or Mountain), 96–97
Eco-boutiques, 309
Edema, 161–162
Elevator Pelvic Pumps, 180
Endorphins, 47, 196
Epidural anesthesia
about, 119–120
losing pain feedback, 200
movement with, 120, 199–200
reducing need for, 187
side effects, 120
Episiotomies, 205–206
Exercise. See also Yoga references
after pregnancy, 243–245
constipation and, 116
dancing, 163, 244
functional training and, 244–245
guidelines, 18–19
lunges, 244

Fasting, 62
Fatigue, 57
Fats, 79–82
healthy sources, 81, 86–87
hydrogenated, partially hydrogenated, 81
importance of, 21, 79–80
indulging in, 81
monounsaturated, 80
omega-3s, 72–73
polyunsaturated, 72–73, 80
recommended daily consumption, 82
saturated, 81
skin care and, 151
to stock, 86–87
TFAs and EFAs, 81
types of, 80–82
unrefined oils, 21–22
Fear
anxiety and, 197
halting labor, 198–199
mantra for (F@$K Everything and Run), 197–199
moving beyond, 199
negative effects of, 197–198
not your friend, 196–197
quelling, by connecting with inner glow, 198–199
Fermenting food, 128
First trimester. See Trimester, first
Flexibility, 92, 202
Folic acid, 24, 71
Food and nutrition. See also Cooking food; Glow foods; Index of Recipes; Vitamins and minerals
boob foods, 235–241
colorful foods, 68
combining foods, 125
complex carbohydrates, 70, 76–77, 130
cravings and, 57–61
fasting and, 62
general guidelines, 63–69
gluten sensitivity, 130–131
greens, 65–67
mindful eating practices, 132–133
mood foods, 225, 227
plant-based focus, 63–64
protein, 69, 74–75, 131–132
quality of food, 64–65
raw foods, 63–64

resources, 308
stopping eating when full, 60
therapeutic vs. comfort foods, 127
vegan lifestyle, xx, 64, 127–128, 310–311
you are what you eat, 64–65
Food dehydrators, 84
Food processors, 84
Forgiveness, 6–7
Formula, for baby, 234–235

Gestational diabetes, 121–122
GLA (gamma linolenic acid) oils, 216
Glimmer detox, 31–33
Glitz detox, 29–31
Glow detox, 33–35
Glow foods
    anticramp, 162
    anti-itch, 160
    antinausea, 54
    antiswelling, 161
    benefits of, 16–17
    blood sugar-balancing, 122
    "boob foods", 235
    for circulation, 163
    complex-carb, 76
    for constipation, 116
    defined, 15–16
    energy-boosting, 57
    examples of, 15–16
    exploring, 15–16
    fun-fatty, 80
    go-to list, 83
    to help you sleep, 111
    lists of, 83, 253
    mineral- and vitamin-rich, 70–72, 74
    mood foods, 225, 227
    omega-rich, 73
    oxidants, antioxidants and, 17
    protein-packed, 74, 132
    reflux-neutralizing, 113
    stocking pantry with, 86–88, 89
    Super-Glow foods, 253
Glow guidelines, 17–25. See also Dairy
    about: conclusion/summary, 251–252
    bathing, 20–21
    cutting out junk food, 23–24
    eating fats and oils, 21–22
    eating sea vegetables/sea salt, 20
    eating super-foods, 22–23
    eating vegetables, 19–20
    eliminating caffeine, 24
    exercising, 18–19
    soy alert, 22
    staying hydrated, 17–18
    taking vitamins, 24–25
Glow Power, 92, 203
Gluten sensitivity, 130–131
Goals
    intention and, 92
    seed, establishing, 46
"God chemical" (DMT), 196, 203
Goddess Squat Series, 139–140, 245
Gratitude, 48, 92, 126, 203, 223
Grounding sequence, 136–138

Hair care, 152, 209
Harper, Tata, 145, 148
Healthcare providers
    birth coaches (doulas), 118, 143, 186–188
    OB/GYN vs. midwife, 120–121. See also Midwives
Herbs, 12, 309
Home
    cleaning, 165–166
    clearing out clutter, 4–5, 47–48
    creating sacred space, 46
    nesting to-dos, 164–166
    revitalizing, repainting, rearranging, 4–5
    surrounding yourself with beauty, 47
Hormones, birth, 194–197. See also specific
    hormones

Induction, 204
Ingredients. See Glow foods; Index of Recipes
Insomnia, 111–113
Insulin
    fasting and, 62
    food intake and, 16, 77, 121–122
    gestational diabetes and, 121–122
    magnesium and, 72
Intention, 92, 126, 201
In Your Life sections, overview of, xxii
Iron, 70–71, 116
Itchy skin, 160–161

Journaling (soul scribing)
    claiming new body, 248
    cleansing limiting beliefs, 9
    getting started, 45–46
    "glowing with the flow", 143
    identifying and eliminating baggage, 8–9
    opening up for birth, 194
    poem to your body parts, 105
    questions to answer, 45–46, 105, 143, 194, 248
Juicers/juice extractors, 84
Junk food, eliminating, 23–24

Kegels, glorified, 179–180
Kitchen. See also Food and nutrition; Glow foods
    tools and equipment, 83–85
Knives, 84
Kroes, Doutzen, 104–105
Krupp, Heidi, 250

Labor. See also Birth; Contractions
    active, 201–202
    birth bag basics, 191–193
    cervix dilation, 168, 200–201
    comfort during, 189–190
    duration of, 201–202
    early, 201
    fear and, 197–199
    hormones of, 195–197
    induction, 204
    moving during, 199–200
    progression, pelvic floor muscles and, 198
    pushing during, 206
    sexual activity before, 166–167, 189. See also
        Orgasms
    transition phase, 202–203
    yoga during, 177–179. See also Yoga (third
        trimester)

Latching challenges, 218–219
Laundry, 165
Leg cramps, 162–163
Leg Drain pose, 181–182
Liver function, 12
Lunch
    about: breastfeeding and, 239
    Glimmer detox, 32, 33
    Glitz detox, 30, 31
    Glow detox, 34
    recipes for. See Index of Recipes
Lunges, 244

Magnesium, 71-72, 113, 116, 162
Mama Glow
    author experience, xvii–xix
    checklist, 208
    defined, xiv
    principles, xxi, xxii, 92–93
    sources of, xiv
    tips for home stretch, 209
Mandolin slicers, 85
Mari, Denise, 145
Mastitis, 219–220
Meditation
    after pregnancy, 250
    breathing and, 94
    clearance movement, 38–39
    food preparation as, 124
    womb-ifestation, 39–40
"Me" time, 250
Midwives
    author experience with, 117
    functions/benefits of, 11, 117–118, 205–206
    slow birth and, 142–143
    using, 117–118, 120–121
    word origin, 11
Mindfulness
    cooking principles, 125–127
    eating practices, 132–133
    labor and, 201
    yoga, 93
Miscarriages, moving past, 11
Mood
    baby blues, PPD and, 222–225
    foods, 225, 227
    mood board for, 194
Morning sickness, 53–55, 300
Mountain Pose, 41, 96–97
Mouth/throat, opening pelvic floor and, 94, 98–100, 167
Music
    birth playlist, 193–194
    sexy, for dancing, 142

Nausea. See Morning sickness
Nesting, details to complete, 164–166
Nut milk bags/cheese cloth, 85

Omega-3s, 72–73
Online communities/resources, 309–310
On the Mat sections, overview of, xxi. See also Yoga references
Opening up
    mouth/throat, sound and, 94, 98–100, 167
    soul scribing for, 194
    yoga for, 93
Orgasms, 46–47, 99, 167, 168, 180, 196
Oxytocin, 189, 195, 201, 202, 203, 215, 232

Pain
    breast/breastfeeding, 216–217, 218–219
    engorgement, 216–217
    fear and, 197–199
    management, 119–120. See also Epidural anesthesia
    natural birth and, 119–120, 169
    transforming into purpose, 169
Pascali-Bonaro, Debra, 206
Patterson, Jodie Baker, 146
PEA (phenylethylamine), 175, 195–196
Pelvic floor muscles
    about, 56–57
    labor progression and, 198
    pelvic pumps and, 179–180
    regenerating after birth, 243
    relaxing, mouth/throat and, 94, 98–100, 167
    sex and, 189
Pelvic pumping, 179–180
Pelvic rolls, 136
Perineum, elasticity of, 189, 202, 206
Phenylethylamine (PEA), 175, 195–196
Pigeon or "Dove Pose", 182–183
Postpartum. See also Breastfeeding
    about: overview of, 213–214
    baby blues and PPD, 222–225
    claiming new body, 243–245
    radical self-care, 247–248
    uni-tasking, 248–249
Postpartum depression (PPD), 223–225
Prayer, 207
Pregnancy
    author experience, xvii–xix
    divinity of, xviii
    preparing for. See Preparing to conceive
    transformational nature of, xix
    "womb-iverse" and, 10–11
Preparing food. See Cooking food
Preparing to conceive, 3–13. See also Clearance, making; Glow guidelines; Prepregnancy detox
    about: overview of, 3–13
    assessing relationships, 5–7
    cleansing limiting beliefs, 8–9
    cleansing your body, 9–10
    clearing out clutter, 4–5, 47–48
    correcting past hurts, 6–7
    Fertili-Tea recipe, 13
    fertility, orgasm and, 47. See also Orgasms
    Glow tips to tune in, 48
    revitalizing your home, 4–5
    unblocking creativity and, 11
    unloading baggage, 7–8
    "womb-iverse" and, 10–11
Prepregnancy detox. See also Glow guidelines
    about, 29; components of, 17; overview of, 12, 17
    herb sources for, 12
    Level I (Glitz), 29–31
    Level II (Glimmer), 31–33
    Level III (Glow), 33–35
    liver function and, 12

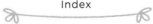

Principles, Mama Glow, xxi, xxii, 92–93
Protein, 69, 74–75, 131–132
P.U.S.H. approach, 206–207

Rashes, 160–161
Reclined Cobbler's Pose, 183
Relationships
    correcting past hurts, 6–7
    forgiveness in, 6–7
    questions to answer about, 5–6
    toxic vs. nurturing, 5–7
    unloading baggage, 7–9
Renewal, planting seeds of, 39

Sacred anatomy, 103–106
Sacred pact, with baby, 53
Sacred space, creating, 46
Sacred Triangle, 97–98
Saline solution boob bath, 222
Salt and salty ingredients, 20, 87
Savory and salty ingredients, 87
Seated goddess posture, 136
Seed goal, 46
Self-care, postpartum, 247–250
Self-love, 105–106
Sensual food preparation, 126–127
Serotonin, 77, 130, 225
Sexual activity, 166–167, 189. See also Orgasms
Sexual organs, 103–104
Shakti Seat (or Cobbler's Pose), 96
Sister circle, 190–191
Skin care
    about: overview of, 146
    body butter, 147
    elasticity of skin, 150–151
    facial masque, 149
    Glow kit and tips, 153
    healthy breakfast for, 148
    ingredients to avoid, 146
    itchiness and rashes, 160–161
    natural products for, 147–150, 151
    product recipes, 147–149, 262
    resources, 310
    scrubs, 148, 149
    stretch marks and, 150–151
Skin-to-skin contact, 207, 222
Sleeplessness, 111–113
Slicer, mandolin, 85
Slings, 227, 306
Slow birth, 142–143
Snacks
    about: breastfeeding and, 239
    Glimmer detox, 32, 33
    Glitz detox, 30
    Glow detox, 34
    recipes for. See Index of Recipes
Soaking food, 128
Soul scribing. See Journaling (soul scribing)
Sound, opening and, 98–100
Soy alert, 22
Space. See also Home
    clearing out clutter, 4–5, 47–48
    holding, 45–48
    sacred, creating, 46
    surrounding yourself with beauty, 47

Sprouting food, 128–129
Squatting, for birth, 200, 205
Standing Cat-Cow Series, 138–139
Standing Flamingo Kicks, 41
Stern, Lyss, 250
Stretch marks, 150–151
Strollers, 306
Style to-dos, 166
Super-foods, 15–16, 22–23
Support
    breastfeeding, 188, 214
    doula for, 118, 143, 186–188
    resources, 305–311
    sister circle, 190–191
Supported Bridge pose, 184
Sweeteners
    complex carbohydrates and, 76–77
    healthy options, 77–78, 88
    insulin levels and, 77
    to stock, 88
    sweet-satisfying healthy recipe, 79
    synthetic, aspartame and, 77
Swelling (edema), 161–162

Theta waves, 168
Thrush, 221–222
To-be list, 249
Tools and equipment, kitchen, 83–85
Triangle Pose, 140–141
Trimester, first. See also Yoga (first trimester)
    about: overview of, 51–52
    baby development, 52
    cravings, 57–61
    eating guidelines, 63–69. See also Food and
        nutrition; Glow foods; Vitamins and minerals
    fasting and, 62
    fatigue, 57
    mama development, 53
    morning sickness, 53–57, 300
    overheating, 53
    sacred anatomy, 104–105
    top three challenges, 53–57
    urination increase, 56–57
Trimester, second. See also Beauty essentials; Yoga
    (second trimester)
    about: overview of, 109
    baby development, 110
    birthing decisions, 117–120
    gestational diabetes and, 121–122
    in the kitchen, 123–133
    mama development, 110–111
    reflux/indigestion/heartburn, 113–115
    sleeplessness, 111–113
    sluggish bowels/constipation, 115–116
    top three challenges, 111–116
Trimester, third. See also Birth; Contractions; Labor;
    Yoga (third trimester)
    about: overview of, 157
    baby development, 158
    brain waves, consciousness and, 168
    defining sister circle, 190–191
    edema, 161–162
    Glow tips for home stretch, 209
    hormone cocktail party, 194–197. See also
        specific hormones

itchy skin and rashes, 160–161
leg cramps, 162–163
mama development, 158–160
Mama Glow checklist, 208
nesting to-dos, 164–166
top three challenges, 160–164
varicose veins, 163–164
Tuning in, 48, 93. *See also* Mindfulness

Uni-tasking, 248–249
Urination, increased, 56–57

Vaginal discharge, 56, 159
Vajroli mudra (pelvic pumping), 179–180
Varicose veins, 163–164
Vegetable peelers, 85
Veins, varicose, 163–164
Vitamin A, 24
Vitamin B (B vitamins)
    for appetite, 54
    B12, 74
    folic acid, 24, 71
    greens and, 66
Vitamin C, 24, 66, 71
Vitamin D, 26
Vitamin E, 24, 66
Vitamin K, 66
Vitamins and minerals. *See also specific vitamins and minerals*
    antioxidant, 17, 24
    greens and, 66
    important ones, 70–72, 74
    vegetables providing, 19
    vitamin primer, 24–25
    when to take, 25

Warrior II, 140, 245
Water
    constipation and, 115, 116
    dehydration issues, 68–69, 162
    flavoring ideas, 69
    intake, importance of, 17–18, 68–69
    plastic bottle precaution, 69
    recommended daily intake, 69
Weaning baby, 239–240
Webb, Veronica, 153
Weight gain, 20, 52, 76, 77, 110, 121–122, 150
Weight loss, after pregnancy, 214, 215, 238
Weight loss, before/during pregnancy, 33, 35
Whackness, weeding out, 11–12
Wodnick, Jill, 125
Womb-ifestation meditation, 39–40
Womb-iverse, 10–11
Writing. *See also* Journaling (soul scribing)
    to most difficult person, 7
    to restore peace, 7

Yoga
    about: overview of this book and, xxi
    after pregnancy, 244–245
    benefits of, 91
    breathing and, 93–95
    flexibility and, 92
    functional training and, 244–245
    Glow Power, 92

gratitude and, 92
grounding sequence, 136–138
intention and, 92
during labor, 177–179
lifestyle resources, 311
Mama Glow principles, 92–93
mindfulness and, 93
opening up, 93, 98–100
postures. *See* Yoga postures
sound, opening and, 98–100
by trimester. *See* Yoga (first trimester); Yoga (second trimester); Yoga (third trimester)
tuning inside and, 93
Yoga (first trimester)
    about: overview of, 91
    affirmations for inner guidance, 100–102
    breathing and, 93–95
    checklist, 102
    making sounds for opening up system, 98–100
    Mama Glow principles, 92–93
    postures, 96–98
Yoga (making clearance plan)
    about, 40–41
    benefits of, 43
    practice, 41–43
Yoga postures
    about: cat, 137; cow, 137; pelvic rolls and, 136; performing, 95; seated goddess posture and, 136
    Awkward Chair Pose, 138
    Boat Pose, 245
    Cat Back/Core Plank, 42
    Child's Pose, 43
    Dove Series, 141
    Downward-Dog Plies, 245
    Downward-Dog Split, 42
    Downward-Facing Dog, 43, 138, 141, 183
    Earth Rooting Pose (Mountain), 96–97
    Goddess Squat Series, 139–140, 245
    Leg Drain, 181–182
    Mountain Pose, 41, 96–97
    Pigeon or "Dove Pose", 182–183
    Reclined Cobbler's Pose, 183
    Sacred Triangle Pose, 97–98
    Shakti Seat (or Cobbler's Pose), 96
    Standing Cat-Cow Series, 138–139
    Standing Flamingo Kicks, 41
    Supported Bridge, 184
    Triangle Pose, 140–141
    Warrior II, 140, 245
Yoga (second trimester), 135–143
    about: overview of, 135
    grounding sequence, 136–138
    sequence of postures, 136–141
    standing poses, 138–141
Yoga (third trimester), 177–184
    benefits during labor, 177–179
    Elevator Pelvic Pumps, 180
    pelvic pumping (vajroli mudra), 179–180
    relax and restore poses, 181–184

Zinc, 72, 114, 131

Acknowledgments

I want to start off with expressing heartfelt gratitude to all those people along my path who made this book possible and/or inspired me along the way. I thank the cosmic mother for ordering my steps and watching over me. I thank my beautiful son, Fulano, for inspiring me along my journey and being the most precious gift I could ever ask for. I thank my mother for being the alchemist she is—crafting my life and giving me every tool possible to succeed. To my father for believing in me. Granny and Grandpa, thank you for your listening ears and wise words. Grandpa Rick, you've been like a father to me and Fulano—thank you for going above and beyond the call of duty. Stacey Rees, my dear midwife who was my glow pilot. Michele Martin, my agent extraordinaire who shared the vision and held it alongside me. To mama Lulu, a.k.a. Louise Hay, for making a way, clearing a path for me to emerge into the light. My editor, Patty Gift, for following her gut and for her TLC. Kris Carr for her sisterhood and coaching me through the book process while it was still in its infancy. Gabrielle Bernstein for being a miracle worker and a spirit guide, and for always elevating my work. Rachel Ash, Danelle Brown, and Haley Binn: thank you for your friendship, holding my hand, and believing in all aspects of the Mama Glow vision. Jill Wodnick and Debra Pascali Bonaro for seeing my strength and supporting my growth as a doula. Carl and Betty: it takes a village . . . thank you for your support. Jeremy Larner for seeing my stardust and having tremendous faith in me. My soul brother, Bryant Terry, for being a shining example for me to follow. Maxwell for your cheerleading and love songs that got me through countless hours of writing. Christy Turlington-Burns, Ricki Lake, and Abby Epstein for your tremendous work and collaboration. Micaela Ezra for the lovely illustrations. I am so grateful to my sisters Nicole Belit, Kate Northrup-Moller, Meggan Watterson, Heidi Krupp, Dana King, Brenda Gloria, Terri Cole, Tigist Selam, Leilani Johnson, Tara Stiles, Anjali Kumar, Pandora Thomas, Marie Forleo, Tsion Ketema, Gigi Parris, Anna Kenney, Denise Albert, Doutzen Kroes, Drena Deniro, Karyn Parsons, Rebecca Minkoff, Saundra Parks, Takeyah Young, Veronica Webb, Jenn Brown, Macha Einbender, Rebecca Walker, Anna Lappé, Rebecca Martin, Natalia Adams, Tata Harper, Audrey Buchanan, Paulina Belle, Cassidy Arkin, and Tracey Henry. Tia and Tamera Mowry for your double dose of glow power! Martin Rowe . . . I did it! To Peg Moline and *Fit Pregnancy* magazine, thank you for standing by me and this book; it's an honor to work with you. To all my clients, past, present, and future who allow me to witness their divine transformation, I love you, I celebrate you. Dr. Richard Ash, Dr. Frank Lipman, and Dr. Mark Hyman, it doesn't get better than you three, thank you for your faith in me and continual uplift. Dr. Christiane Northrup, my iconic mentor, you are a priestess, thank you for your wisdom and grace. The light in me bows to each of you.

ABOUT THE AUTHOR

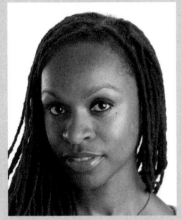

Latham Thomas is a maternity lifestyle maven, wellness and birth coach, and yoga teacher on the vanguard of transforming the maternal wellness movement. A graduate of Columbia University and The Institute for Integrative Nutrition, Latham is the founder of Mama Glow – a holistic maternity lifestyle brand helping women to explore their creative edge through optimal wellbeing. Her practice provides support to pre/postnatal women along their journey to motherhood offering culinary and nutritional services, yoga and birth-coaching services.

Latham strives to educate, empower and inspire her clients during pregnancy and help them look and feel their most radiant. She is co-founder of the Mama Glow Film Festival, (www.mamaglowfilmfest.com) a platform for maternal advocacy through film and philanthropy, and she launched the Mama Glow Salon Series (www.mamaglow salonseries.com), a platform for birthing conversations around cocktails, panels and discussions.

Bridging the gap between optimal wellness, spiritual growth and radical self-care, Latham Thomas is emerging as the go-to guru for modern holistic lifestyle for women during pregnancy and beyond! A sought-after nutrition and lifestyle expert, she has been featured in the *New York Daily News, New York Post, Time Out New York, AM New York, New York Family* magazine, *Vogue.com, Whole Living, VegNews, Fit Pregnancy,* and on the cover of *Experience Life* magazine. She lives in New York City with her son Fulano and their turtle Climby. Latham is helping to green the planet one belly at a time.

To learn more about Latham Thomas, visit her online at www.mamaglow.com, and stay in the glow on Facebook (Latham Thomas-Mama Glow) and on Twitter (@GlowMaven).

www.mamaglow.com

333

SHARE THE GLOW!

Were you inspired, touched, motivated, and uplifted by Mama Glow? If so, I would like to invite you to be a part of the movement to help spread the glow power. My mission is to empower women with this message and spark their inner light. I would love your help!

- **Send us an email or video testimonial.** I love hearing your glow tips, experiences, and feelings: info@mamaglow.com

- **Visit our website and join our mailing list:** www.mamaglow.com

- **Tweet from the mountain tops!** Send a tweet sharing the book using @GlowMaven and #MamaGlowBook in your message. Posting quoteables from the book are helpful, too!

- **Buy this book for someone else.** Give it to a woman you know, leave it in an OB/GYN office, or donate it to your local library.

- **Post your glow tips on Facebook.** Are you practicing some of the methods in the book and have some of your own glow tips to share? Post on our Facebook page.

- **Post a review online.** Visit bookseller sites like Amazon and B&N, and post your review of the book. If you have a blog, post a review there as well.

- **Start a Mama Glow support posse.** Find a friend or group of friends you can do the book with; share your dreams, visions, and goals; and support and hold each other accountable.

Hay House Titles of Related Interest

YOU CAN HEAL YOUR LIFE, the movie, starring Louise L. Hay & Friends
(available as a 1-DVD program and an expanded 2-DVD set)
Watch the trailer at: **www.LouiseHayMovie.com**

THE SHIFT, the movie,
starring Dr Wayne W. Dyer
(available as a 1-DVD program and an expanded 2-DVD set)
Watch the trailer at: **www.DyerMovie.com**

BABY TO TODDLER MONTH BY MONTH, by Simone Cave and Dr Caroline Fertleman

COPING WITH TWO: A Stress-free Guide to Managing a New Baby When You Have Another Child, by Simone Cave and Dr Caroline Fertleman

CRAZY SEXY KITCHEN: 150 Plant-Empowered Recipes to Ignite a Mouthwatering Revolution, by Kris Carr

HEART THOUGHTS: A Daily Guide to Finding Inner Wisdom, by Louise L. Hay

MEDIDATING: Meditations for Fearless Romance, by Gabrielle Bernstein

MOM ENERGY: A Simple Plan to Live Fully Charged, by Ashley Koff, RD, and Kathy Kaehler

RIGHT TIME BABY: The Complete Guide to Later Motherhood by Claudia Spahr

YOU CAN CREATE AN EXCEPTIONAL LIFE, by Louise Hay and Cheryl Richardson

All of the above are available at your local bookstore,
or may be ordered by contacting Hay House (see next page).

We hope you enjoyed this Hay House book. If you'd like to receive
our online catalogue featuring additional information on
Hay House books and products, or if you'd like to find out
more about the Hay Foundation, please contact:

Hay House UK, Ltd., 292B Kensal Rd., London W10 5BE
Phone: 0-20-8962-1230 • *Fax:* 0-20-8962-1239
www.hayhouse.co.uk • www.hayfoundation.org

Published and distributed in the United States by: Hay House, Inc., P.O. Box 5100, Carlsbad,
CA 92018-5100 • *Phone:* (760) 431-7695 or (800) 654-5126
Fax: (760) 431-6948 or (800) 650-5115• www.hayhouse.com®

Published and distributed in Australia by: Hay House Australia Pty. Ltd., 18/36 Ralph St.,
Alexandria NSW 2015 • *Phone:* 612-9669-4299 • *Fax:* 612-9669-4144 • www.hayhouse.com.au

Published and distributed in the Republic of South Africa by: Hay House SA (Pty), Ltd.,
P.O. Box 990, Witkoppen 2068 • *Phone/Fax:* 27-11-467-8904 • www.hayhouse.co.za

Published in India by: Hay House Publishers India, Muskaan Complex, Plot No. 3, B-2, Vasant
Kunj, New Delhi 110 070 • *Phone:* 91-11-4176-1620 • *Fax:* 91-11-4176-1630 • www.hayhouse.co.in

Distributed in Canada by: Raincoast, 9050 Shaughnessy St., Vancouver, B.C. V6P 6E5 •
Phone: (604) 323-7100 • *Fax:* (604) 323-2600 • www.raincoast.com

Take Your Soul on a Vacation

Visit **www.HealYourLife.com**® to regroup, recharge,
and reconnect with your own magnificence.
Featuring blogs, mind-body-spirit news, and
life-changing wisdom from Louise Hay and friends.

Visit **www.HealYourLife.com** today!

Free e-newsletters
from Hay House, the Ultimate
Resource for Inspiration

Be the first to know about Hay House's dollar deals, free downloads, special offers, affirmation cards, giveaways, contests, and more!

 Get exclusive excerpts from our latest releases and videos from *Hay House Present Moments*.

 Enjoy uplifting personal stories, how-to articles, and healing advice, along with videos and empowering quotes, within *Heal Your Life*.

 Have an inspirational story to tell and a passion for writing? Sharpen your writing skills with insider tips from *Your Writing Life*.

Sign Up Now!

Get inspired, educate yourself, get a complimentary gift, and share the wisdom!

http://www.hayhouse.com/newsletters.php

Visit www.hayhouse.com to sign up today!

 HAY HOUSE

HAYHOUSE RADIO))) *radio for your soul®*

HealYourLife.com